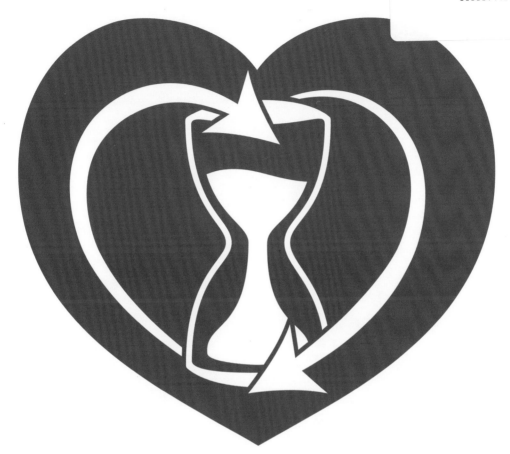

The Body Rescue
MAINTENANCE
Plan

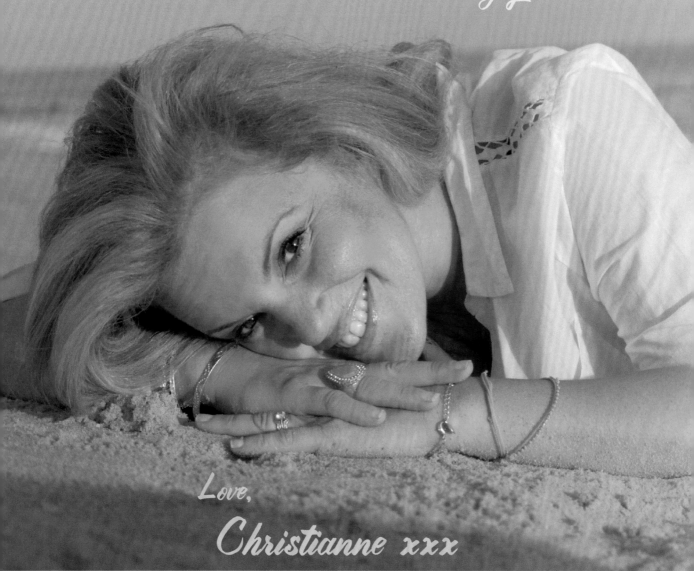

This book is yours for life – a life plan of happiness with nutrition to feed your body, exercise to tone your muscles, and mindset to nurture your soul. Enjoy!

Love,

Christianne xxx

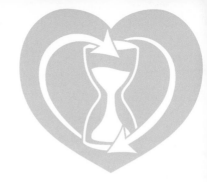

Thank you

With special thanks to my helpers Louise Harper, Kelly Ballard, Sarah Magee and Anne Wolff.

Paul Magee and Andres Le Sauvage for the fantastic photography.

Louise Banks for the beautiful artwork.

Julie Lewthwaite for the editing.

And everyone who has helped me on my amazing journey.

About Christianne

Christianne Wolff is a multi-award-winning celebrity trainer, expert in weight loss and healing, and author of three books, *The Body Rescue Plan*, *The Body Rescue Detox Recipe Book* and *The Body Rescue Maintenance Plan*.

Christianne writes several columns for the national press and appears in the international media every week.

Christianne owns The Body Rescue Fitness Slimming Clubs, which run all over the UK, and runs her Body Rescue Retreats worldwide.

For more information go to:
www.thebodyrescueplan.com

PUBLISHED BY
Body Rescue Ltd
Saxeway Business Centre,
Chartridge Lane,
Chartridge.
Bucks.
HP5 2SH
07977 714 791
www.thebodyrescueplan.com

ISBN 978-1-5262-0480-6

DISCLAIMER
Before starting this programme you may wish to seek medical advice from a doctor and get permission to start The body rescue maintenance plan. The advice and instruction in The body rescue maintenance plan does not replace any medical procedure. Christianne Wolff disclaims any liability or loss. The body rescue maintenance plan is not recommended if you are pregnant.

CONTENTS

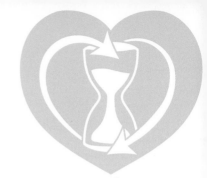

FOREWORD

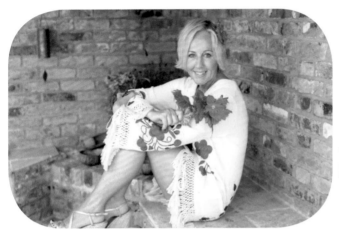

"I am so pleased that Christianne has released another wonderful informative book on healthy eating, mindset, diet and lifestyle. She always has such bountiful energy and a positive mind that just turning the pages of The Body Rescue Maintenance Plan made me feel better!

Body Rescue is a way of living, educating yourself about yourself, and I highly recommend Christianne's plans to achieve all your goals in health & fitness for a better way of living and weight loss!

I lost weight on The Body Rescue Plan, gained more energy and felt like I jump-started my whole system, mind and body.

I found Christianne's mentoring and encouragement to eat well and stay fit so inspiring, that I feel healthier and better than ever before and continue to do so on The Maintenance Plan. I am meeting more and more women my age who are suffering from fatigue and weight gain and feel this is the perfect plan for them.

Christianne's authenticity in how she lives her life and her enthusiasm to share her knowledge for a better way of life is invaluable."

Shirlie Kemp

QUOTES *from the* PRESS

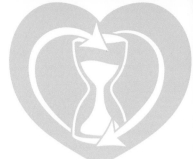

"Hone your body to get an A list physique, with this total body workout."
HEALTH AND FITNESS MAGAZINE

"My attitude towards healthy eating and exercise has undergone a life-changing turnaround, due to Body Rescue."
YOUR AMERSHAM MAGAZINE - MIMI HARKER OBE

"Christianne shows ways to 24/7 your fat burn."
WOMEN'S HEALTH

"Christianne Wolff has some amazingly healthy recipes and shows how comfort foods can be healthy."
THE DAILY MAIL

"Christianne Wolff shows how the Duke of Cambridge adapts impressive yoga moves."
THE TIMES

"Award-winning author Christianne Wolff shows how to rev up your metabolism."
YOUR FITNESS MAGAZINE

"Christianne reveals surprising reasons why you are not losing weight."
WOMEN'S WEEKLY MAGAZINE

"Celebrity trainer Christianne Wolff shows how to improve your digestion with yoga."
THE DAILY MIRROR

TESTIMONIALS

The Allisons

This lovely family lost over 12 stone between them on The Body Rescue Plan and have continued to lose weight on the Maintenance Plan or kept it off since, following the simple rules.

You can watch their inspiring video on our website:
www.thebodyrescueplan.com/success-stories/

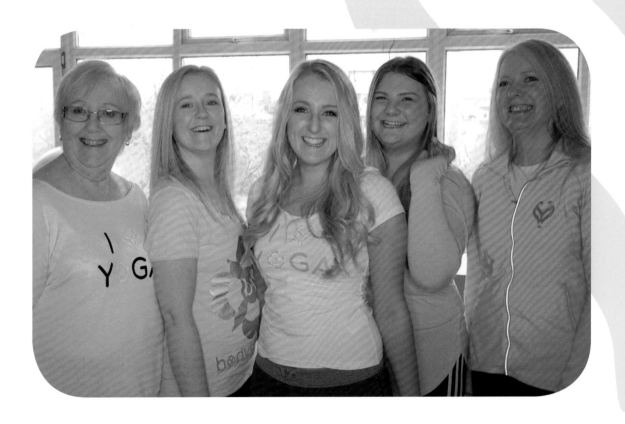

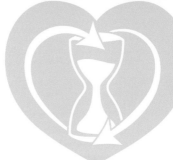

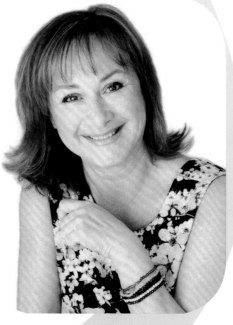

Ariane Poole

CELEBRITY MAKE UP ARTIST

"I can't praise the Body Rescue Plan and Christianne Wolff highly enough.

It has been a game changer for me. Having gone through the menopause I couldn't get rid of my extra weight around my middle. I am in the public eye, appearing on TV and giving talks all over the world about make-up and looking great. My weight was really getting me down! I tried EVERYTHING!!

Nothing worked until I tried the Body Rescue Plan in September 2014. I lost 21lbs. in 12 weeks. This is a lifestyle, NOT a diet! It helps you change your attitude to food. Educates you (in a nice way) how the food we eat has a huge impact on our body and mind.

I've kept the weight off for nearly a year now, including the indulgences of Christmas and Birthdays. I'm doing the Body Rescue Plan Maintenance online now; the recipes are so delicious, Christianne's support is amazing. I am very happy, I am me, but better! I would HIGHLY recommend this to everyone. You have nothing to lose but weight! It works on the person as a whole!"

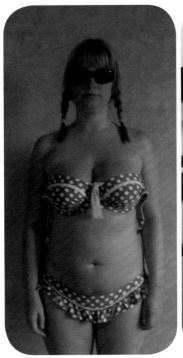
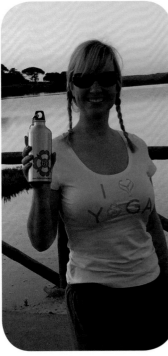

Catherine Huntley

TV PRESENTER

" I'm now two years on from where I started The Body Rescue Plan. I started as a size 16 and went down to a 10. I'm thrilled to say I'm currently a 10. I fluctuate between a 10 and a 12 and I think that's down to the fact that I am totally in control of my food now. If I have weddings or other special events in the diary where I want to have a few glasses of fizz, a slice of cake or even a takeaway, I can. I believe the maintenance plan has enabled me to keep my weight and health steady and consistent. Many diets get you down to your goal weight, but what then?

Often, and I speak from experience, we just put all the pre-diet weight back on. With lots of diets, losing weight isn't necessarily the hardest part - it's keeping it off. Christianne really cares about people and it shows in the maintenance plan she has devised. What's great is my two adult children have also come to embrace this healthier lifestyle. We genuinely enjoy coming up with new recipe ideas together, based on what we've learnt, and going for walks to get exercise. I've noticed a real shift in the way the world eats and how they care for their bodies. This means shopping for healthier ingredients has become far easier than when I started the plan. I'm proud to say I still reap the benefits to this day and am so glad Christianne, and all her knowledge, came into my life."

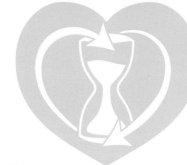

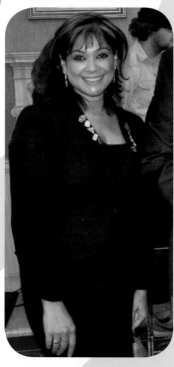
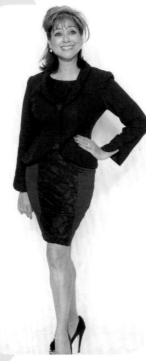

Mimi Harker OBE

" I decided to take my life into my own hands and do The Body Rescue Plan. Before I did this plan I was starting to become despondent with myself. My weight started to creep on and on a little bit more. Every year I noticed my waist getting bigger inch by inch. All of a sudden I was a size 14 from a size 6 and I thought to myself, is it too late to do something about this? And then my friend told me about The Body Rescue Plan and WOW! What a difference I am seeing now.

The best part for me, and the most encouraging, was that my weight came off so quickly in the first 2 weeks. You get to my age, which is middle-aged, and you think that's the middle-aged spread and its never going to go and they tell you it happens. So when I saw the weight come off I was really encouraged. At first I was a bit skeptical - is that really what the scales were saying? But it did work and I felt amazing and it made me keep going. The most incredible thing is that I have lost 6 inches around my waist, I was 31 inches and now I am 25! Which is what I was when I got married 27 years ago.

The Body Rescue Plan has changed my life in so many ways. I am so much happier. When I first read the book I thought it won't work for me because nothing else has. But it really changes your mindset and helps you with healthy eating. Even my husband's portly tummy has gone totally flat now."

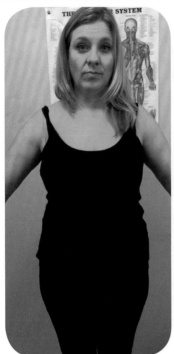 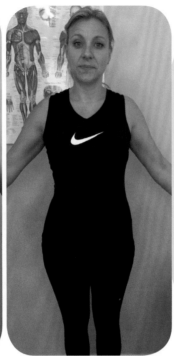

Liz Franklin

"I got to the end of 2015 feeling tired, fat, lethargic and very unhealthy. Another dry January was not going to be a solution to how I was feeling, so I embarked on a 12 week Body Rescue Plan with Christianne. If I couldn't take 12 weeks of my life out for me and the sake of my health, then I really did think that I was beyond help.

Yes, I wanted to lose weight and feel slimmer, but I also wanted to make a lifestyle change that was easy, doable day-to-day and would fit in with my very busy life. I work as a self-employed PA, which is demanding, as well as running around after my 7 year old. Having a glass of wine every night and eating late was a general routine, but things had to change otherwise the scales would be going up and up.

Within the first week, the support and the daily encouragement I received from Christianne spurred me on to really embrace the simplicity of her plan. The first week I thought was going to be hard, but how wrong was I? No calorie counting, no measuring, no fancy recipes or weird foods to eat. Just good simple, basic but tasty food ideas, and plenty of it. I lost 8lbs in the first two weeks and loved discovering new ways to cook healthy and delicious food. My time in the kitchen halved, my energy levels went through the roof and I began to feel like a whole new person very literally overnight.

By week 6 I had lost over a dress size and was nearly on my way to losing 2. The body mass was melting off me and I actually wanted to exercise!

The plan is not like other weight loss plans - its just good, clean living which rejuvenates your body instantly. The exercises were fun and I loved Christianne's inspirational ideas to stay on track every day. No sugar cravings, no longing for all the guilty pleasures we crave for daily, and an energy that I've not felt in decades. Not to mention the sound sleep I was having night after night.

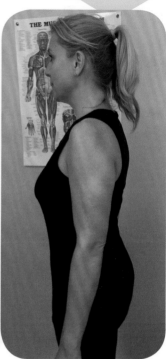

I'm now on the Maintenance Plan - I shop, cook and eat better, I feel slim and trim, I have had so many compliments from friends and family about my 'glow' - its all down to Christianne's incredible support and The Body Rescue Plan.

I weighed 12 stone 8 pounds and was a size 16. I am now 10 stone 12 pounds and a size 12. Only an inch or two to go until I can fit into that size 10 LBD I've bought as my goal prize!

One very happy customer!"

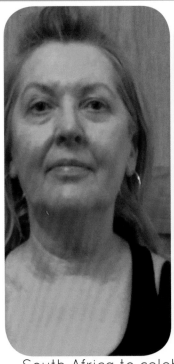
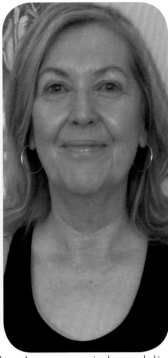

Anne Dawson
TV PRESENTER

" What is the toughest part of losing weight? Yes, as we all know ... it's keeping it off!!

Well, I'm thrilled to say that after completing the original Body Rescue programme ... I'm now 3 months down the road and all still looking good!! And do you know what? Christianne has so cracked the system that it's actually easy!!!

Let me back up slightly ... just before Christmas I went to South Africa to celebrate a special wedding anniversary. Fabulous holiday ... but I spent most of it hiding under large, loose tent-like clothing as I was at my heaviest ever!! I already knew that Christianne's programme worked as I share a dressing room with Catherine Huntley at QVC and she has had amazing success ... and kept the weight off, too. So upon putting away the Christmas decorations (plus a week or so to finish the odd mince pie here and there), I decided to bite the bullet and go for it.

Check out the photo's ... week one, 15th January, and then week ten of the twelve week programme!! I shed 16 pounds, but it wasn't actually the scales that surprised me the most. I dropped 13 inches just between my waist and my hips, and a whopping great 13% body fat!!!!! My whole appearance changed and I have never had so many compliments in my life.

Well, 12 weeks later and another 5 pounds lighter (without really trying) I am more convinced than ever that I have been given the winning combination that unlocks the toughest part of dieting ... keeping the weight off! The secret? A total life change in your eating habits!! Like so many, I've lost weight before and then put it all back on, and more, but with the eating plans and delicious recipes that Christianne advocates, it is so much easier. I am positively addicted to her broccoli soup (who'd have thought I'd ever say that!!). And her 'treats' are so yummy......I've had afternoon tea (herbal, of course) loads of times with her scone recipe, and my friends have been amazed!! I'm even making my own chocolate these days!!!

But for me the real litmus test on a maintenance plan is what happens when you go on holiday or there's a night out or another celebration? Well, I've had 3 trips to Italy since week 10, along with many meals out, birthday celebrations, etc., and like I said, I'm still ahead of the game.

I honestly reckon that when you're maintaining your weight, it's what you do most of the time that counts. And let's face it, you're only going to do something the majority of the time if you enjoy it.
Previously at this stage of any eating plan I've tended to feel like a stretched elastic band waiting to ping and then end up just going back to my old ways ... but no more!!

Christianne has revealed the mystery and given us the method, the tools and all the encouragement we need to succeed ... and stay there!! I know it sounds so 'cliched' to say something is positively life changing, but truly, that is precisely what this is. I feel better at 56 years old than I did in my forties.

Try it! You won't look back!!"

INTRODUCTION

The Body Rescue Plan was devised and drawn from my knowledge, from all the courses I have ever been on, from all the books I have read, and from all the qualifications I have achieved over the last twenty years. But far more importantly than that, The Body Rescue Plan was born from my intuitive energy, a guidance I use with my clients to drive me to get the right results for them.

I don't automatically trust everything I read and everything I learn – it has to be proven to me through trying it for myself, trying it with my clients, and having that 'feeling' that it works. I have also been in the fitness industry long enough to realise that everything that seems to get 'scientifically proven' usually gets 'disproven' a few years later. We are still relatively young in the diet and fitness industry, it's really only since the 1980s that medical science took any notice of fitness and diets, and really only since the 1950s that people took up exercise and 'healthy' eating plans.

The diet and fitness industry is worth billions, and most companies that pump out diet and fitness products unfortunately don't care if you are actually healthy and will live long and be happy, they are just jumping on the bandwagon to make a quick buck. So for me it was really important to bring out a book that makes you think about how you really feel, not just another book about counting calories and the slimmest person wins. It's about understanding why you consume, why you use food as a crutch, why you are addicted to foods that make you feel negative, and really the ultimate aim of any goal should be to be happier. If starving yourself, and working out all the hours of the day, and being obsessed with the numbers on the scales is not making you happier you will ultimately put that weight back on again. The Body Rescue Plan is about tuning into YOU. Who are you? Why do you behave in a certain way? How can you make changes to be happier and healthier? It's about eating foods that make you feel amazing, that give you your energy back, that feed your cells to become abundantly healthy and vibrant and slim.

The Body Rescue Plan is a twelve-week course that detoxes your body and makes you realise what foods agree with you and what foods do not. It teaches you how to cook nutrient-dense food in a delicious and easy way. It teaches you to understand your mindset and to use the power of meditation to heal your old wounds. It teaches you to use yoga to lengthen and

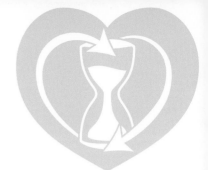

strengthen your body, and it teaches you to use some high-powered exercises that are simple enough to do anywhere, quick to complete, and get you the results you are looking for.

The Body Rescue Maintenance Plan is a plan for life. Following your initial twelve-week journey you can now follow this really simple plan to keep you feeling amazing, finely tuned and evolving for the rest of your life. We still follow the same principles as in The Body Rescue Plan, with the nutrition, the exercise and the mindset as below.

The Maintenance Eating Plan

This is the same as following week six of The Body Rescue Plan, while also having one or two days off per week. In this book I teach you how to understand how much time to have off the plan, how not to get addicted to foods again, and how you can maintain your weight for life in a controlled yet free way. I also have some delicious recipes with monthly eating plans to suit everyone. There are vegetarian, gluten-free, summer and winter plans, recipes, and shopping lists, too.

The Maintenance Mindset Plan

Your mind now will be far stronger and more in tune with your body and you will just need a maintenance mindset plan to follow – some simple exercises to keep you relaxed and calm, happy and grounded. We also develop gratitude a little further, as gratitude is very powerful.

The Maintenance Exercise Plan

I have developed some new, exciting exercises for you in The Body Rescue Maintenance Plan. They're still structured as they were in The Body Rescue Plan, with interval training, resistance training, cardio, abs and yoga, as I feel all these exercises give you the most rounded training performance and the most toned physique in a relatively short period of time. The exercises are also really easy to do and they still require no equipment, so fitting them into your life is simple, you can do them anywhere, there's very little space needed and exercise doesn't take up your entire day.

CHAPTER 1

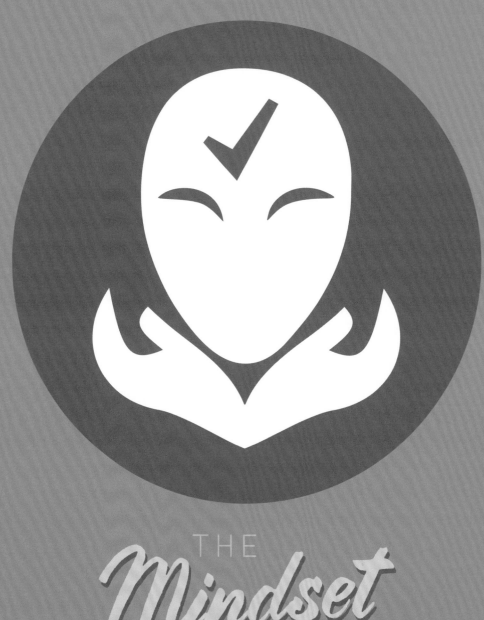

THE
Mindset

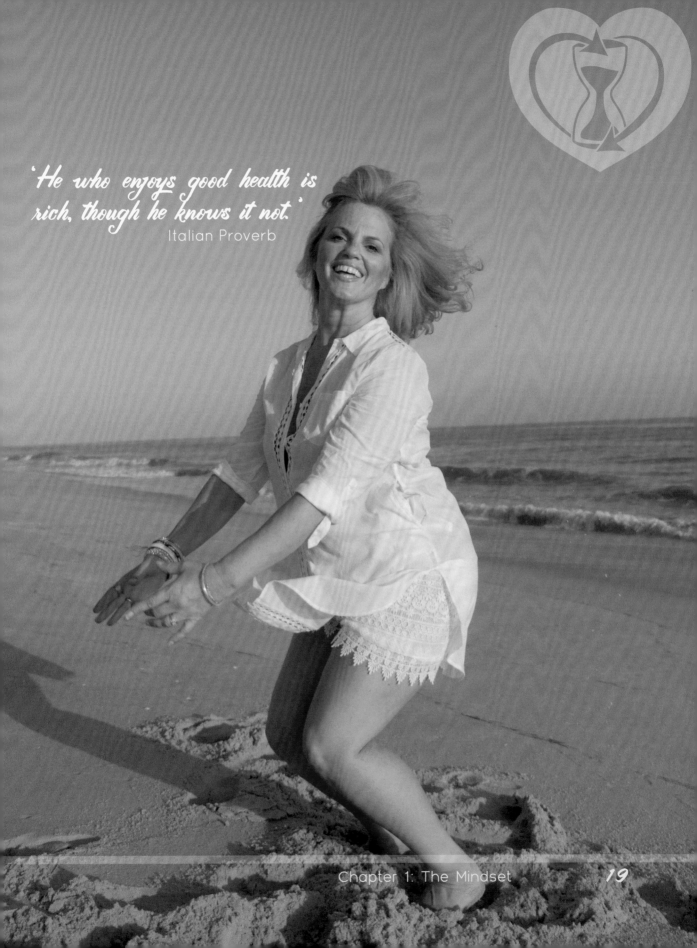

'He who enjoys good health is rich, though he knows it not.'
Italian Proverb

Chapter 1: THE Mindset

Gratitude

In my book The Body Rescue Plan we focused a lot on the mindset, because I really wanted you to have the groundwork there, the foundation laid down first before going back to 'normal' eating. You will have gone on a beautiful journey of self-discovery, ups and downs, ins and outs. You will have worked through your trigger points and limiting beliefs and realised that a few more came up on the way for you to work through again, only to come out the other side winning!

At this point on starting the maintenance plan I want to keep the mindset work as simple as possible for you. The whole point of the maintenance plan is that you have done the hard work and now you can be as free as a bird and enjoy your fabulous new body and health, while also realising that your mind is like a muscle and still needs a regular workout to stay strong.

So, just a few ground rules to think about.

First of all, where do you want to go from here?

Some of my clients, once they have achieved the desired weight loss and got really fit, discover they suddenly have a hunger for a lot more – so once the twelve-week plan is completed they then set another, bigger goal, like doing a triathlon, or a marathon, or taking up a new sport, or joining a cycling club. If you feel you want to take your body one step further that is absolutely brilliant, but it's not essential and I have not included the training or mindset for those goals.

If you want to reach further than just maintaining your body, what I would suggest is you revisit your trigger points and limiting beliefs regularly, as with every goal you set and achieve, new limiting beliefs will come up and then you will triumph over those, too.

Setting new goals is fantastic and a great way to stay on track, so you don't get bored and you always feel like you are achieving something. That's why

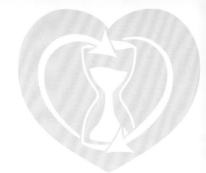

I have changed the exercise regime for this plan every two months, so you don't become stagnant. Even as part of the maintenance plan you can set yourself goals within the cardio section, maybe by doing something you haven't tried before. I am always amazed at the amount of clients I have had who can't swim or cycle. But once they get into it, they love it!

Take my client, Paul Field. *(Read his testimonial in The Body Rescue Plan.)* He could barely swim and had never cycled, and after losing a few stone with me he said he wanted to set a new goal – because he didn't have much time I suggested he use the Boris Bikes in London.

So, he got the train into London and first of all cycled a fairly short distance, and eventually a longer distance, and then cycled thirty minutes from the Tube to his place of work, and back again. It took some organisation with clothes, etc., but he did it most days.

The next stage was for him to buy his own fold-up bike, which he took on the train with him, and again he cycled to and from the Tube station. Then he got so into cycling, he bought another super-dooper lightweight bike and even cycled from where he lived into work, which was seventy miles there and back. After that he was an addict.

I then taught him to swim – after which he did a few mini-triathlons, triathlons, and now he does Iron Man Triathlons! Oh, and he is in his forties and had never worked out before he met me.

If you are setting new goals, remember to still do your goal-setting meditations, as these really help keep you on track.

Planning is still important, especially as you have reached your goal now – you still want to keep things exciting, still want to try new recipes (don't just stick to the same old favourites), planning where you will fit your workouts in and making sure that spot does not get prioritised with anything else.

I would say there are two main reasons people fail at keeping their weight off and maintaining their fitness levels, and they are because they stopped planning and they stopped being thankful. So don't take this for granted – just do it each week. After doing The Body Rescue Plan this will probably be second nature by now, so it will be easy for you to carry on with it. But again, make sure that you add a little bit of spice each week. Do not always do exactly the same run, or cycle the same route, or go to the same Zumba class – mix it up and keep it interesting and plan plan plan. Use my diary printout on www.thebodyrescueplan.com, or use my Body Rescue app to mark down your diary each week.

The attitude of gratitude

What I want you to focus on mainly, though, is gratitude, because without having a sense of feeling how grateful you are for your amazing body, and how happy you are to feel so good, you will start to take your new body and mind for granted and then start focusing again on things that are wrong with your body.

You may have even started doing it already. Perhaps you were once one or two or three stone heavier, or more, and your ultimate dream may have been to lose all that weight, and now you have lost all that weight you may have gone through a euphoric feeling only now to be dissatisfied again. Perhaps now you want to look like a supermodel, or want a six-pack. And this is fine – as humans we constantly want to evolve and it's far better to want to evolve than sit on the couch with a bucket of ice cream and get more and more unhealthy, but with every step on the evolutionary plain you take, you must always be grateful for what you have already.

What (if anything) are you still unhappy with about your body?

How can you improve this?

What are you grateful for in your body?

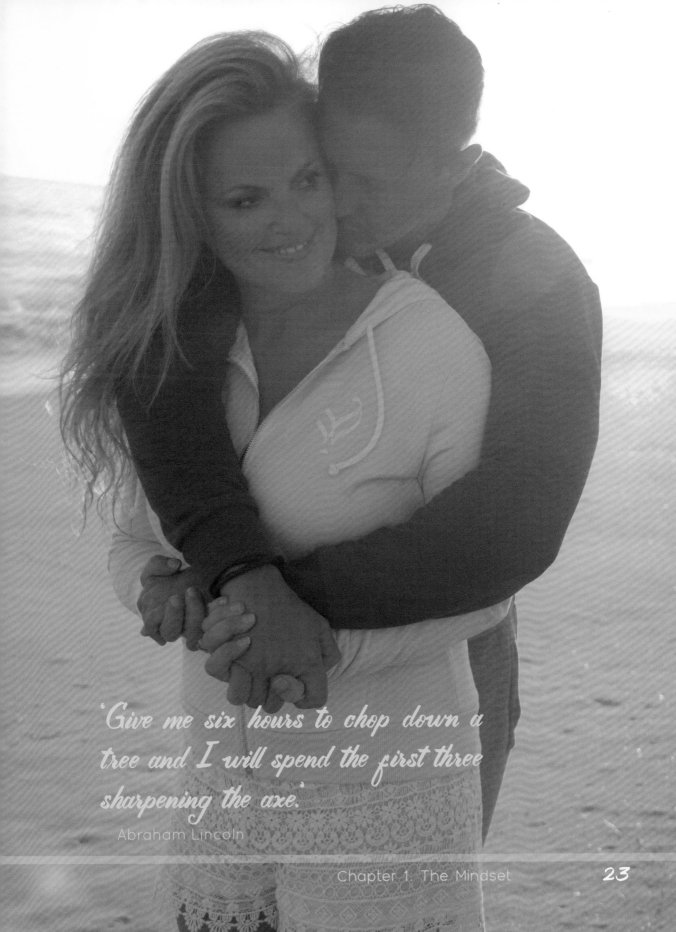

'Give me six hours to chop down a tree and I will spend the first three sharpening the axe.'

Abraham Lincoln

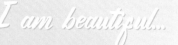

I am beautiful...

My heart beats
My blood flows
My cells grow
My skin glows

My heart beats
My mouth tastes
My love has no haste
My liver removes waste

My heart beats
My words sing
My pancreas releases insulin

My heart beats
My bones protect
My brain sends messages
which I reflect

My arms carry
My ears listen
My hair is my mane, it grows
and glistens

My womb reproduces
My body digests
My breasts feed
My eyebrows hold sweat

My bones protect
My tongue tastes
My joints lever
My mind races

My soul has passion
My soul feels love
My soul sends healing from the
sky above

If every day I did consider
How incredible it is that my
body is still here
I would perhaps not crave for
more
But be thankful My heart beats,
one day more.

Christianne Wolff

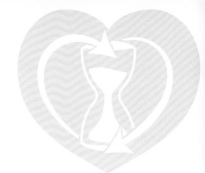

Your body is incredible. You have trillions of cells working for you every day, without you asking them to. All your senses let you enjoy the magnificence of life, and the magic! Your limbs help you carry, create, run ... Your heart keeps all your organs working and alive. Do you ever just stop and thank your body for working so hard for you?

Your body's primary purpose is to heal itself. That is all it wants to do for you – heal itself whilst you are awake, or whilst you are asleep. Whether you offer it nourishment or throw toxicity and negativity at it, it will still strive to heal you.

I often hear the words, 'Damn you, body, for not working properly,' when someone is ill, or injured or down. But if you just stopped for one minute and said, 'Thank you so much, body, for healing me,' you would instantly feel better and you'd improve far more quickly.

I remember once when I had pneumonia, I was really sick in bed and feeling very sorry for myself. I was also quite scared as I have never felt so close to death before, and not being able to breathe certainly gave me a huge appreciation of how amazing it is to get a clear breath, something we take for granted every day. As I was lying in bed one day I decided to surf the Internet for health and nutrition documentaries, all of which were fascinating. But there was one line that really struck a chord with me whilst I was watching one of them, and that was the one that stated **'Your body's primary purpose is to heal itself, that is all it wants to do for you'**. I felt so emotional when I heard those words – from feeling like I was dying, I suddenly felt a rush of love pour out of my heart to my body, thanking it so much for fighting off the pneumonia as hard as it possibly could – it was doing everything it could for me, and from that point on I got better. I actually felt instantly more healed.

So next time you get ill or injured thank your body for swelling up on you – that's its way of protecting you; or thank it for showing you pain – that's its way of protecting you; or thank it for perhaps slowing your digestion down whilst it protects your vital organs. Protection is its aim, and any pain you may feel is because it wants to heal you.

Do you feel any pain or injury at the moment?

How can you thank your body for feeling this way? How is it protecting you?

What I would like you to do now is put a photo of yourself on a piece of paper, or on your computer screen, or wherever it feels good for you – I also have this facility on my new app and in my gratitude diary, if you prefer to use that. You can go here:

www.thebodyrescueplan/app   **www.thebodyrescueplan/gratitudediary**

By your photo I would like you to write what you appreciate about your body today.

Start with ten things, and every day I want you to add one more. This is so healing for the body, and amazing through good times and bad. When you want to grow, it allows you to focus on the amazing things your body has triumphed through and when you are feeling slower, it allows you to realise just how incredible your body is every day, even without the bigger achievements.

The more you focus on being thankful for what you have, the more you will appreciate it and keep it. The more you chastise yourself and ridicule your body, the more you will lose it. Just think about if you talked to someone else the way you sometimes talk to yourself. Imagine going up to someone and saying, 'I think you are really fat and worthless because you still have a muffin top, despite losing all that weight; I think you don't look as beautiful as a model so all that work was pointless; I think that because you can't get into a size ten pair of jeans you shouldn't even think about attracting someone in your life.'

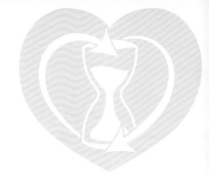

If you said that to someone else they would probably go and top themselves! They would feel terrible, no matter how much self-confidence they had, and more than likely they would think, *What's the point? I will just eat a load of junk food again.*

So, if you made someone else feel like that, why wouldn't you make yourself feel like that, too? Even just sitting here typing those words has made my whole vibration change. After writing such loving words, the vibration of those negative words affects me and you, whether reading, writing or saying them. So stop! Love yourself and write down every day what you are thankful for in your amazing body.

Start today with your top ten!

1 Thank you, body, for ...

2 ....

3 ....

4 ....

5 ....

6 ....

7 ....

8 ....

9 ....

10 ....

Place a photo here!

'For what we are about to receive, may the Lord make us truly thankful.'

I would like you also to extend your gratitude to the food you eat. Often we can feel that somehow we are missing out if we can't have certain foods or drinks. Of course we know now this is just in our mindset and that the real 'missing out' is lack of energy, the ageing skin, the overweight body, the depressed mind, the stiff joints, etc. – these are the reasons we really miss out, if we eat junk foods and drinks every day.

Saying grace was part of most household rituals no less than a hundred years ago; now it seems a dying tradition.

In Jewish communities it's called Birkat Hamazon.

In Christian communities it's called Grace.

Hindus use the Bhagavad Gita prayer.

In Japan it is customary to put one's hands together and say 'Itadakimasu', (いただきます), 'I humbly receive', before eating a meal.

In Korea, they say 'Jal meokgesseumnida', (잘 먹겠습니다), 'I will eat well'.

Some Christian religions also have prayers to say after they have eaten, too, giving thanks again.

Whether you are religious or not, whether you are thanking God, or the universe or just yourself, you can still appreciate and be mindful of what is going in your mouth to heal you and give you energy and stimulate your senses. Eating is one of the greatest pleasures in life, and should be felt that way.

So all I would love you to do is before each meal and before each snack give thanks. I even do this whilst shopping, it makes shopping far more exciting if you touch and feel each fruit and vegetable and think about how wonderful the colours are, and the smells and textures of all these delicious

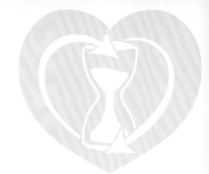

foods that will be making you healthier and happier and just say thank you – even to the piece of fruit for growing just for you.

As well as food, think about how amazing water is for you. Everything on the planet relies on water to keep itself alive. We are made up of about sixty per cent water, it is part of us integrally.

Dr Masaru Emoto wrote a book about the effect on water when you play it soft music, when you swear or shout at it, and when you subject it to other environments, and then took a series of photos of the molecules in the water as a result. The results were astounding, and speak for themselves. The water molecules when shouted at and abused were very ugly and fractured. The water molecules that were blessed, spoken to with love and had soft music played to them were beautiful. If you bless the water and food you eat, this will become part of you – you are mainly water!

As well as this I have recorded some gratitude meditations for you to keep you really strong with your gratitude.

Please go here to download :

www.thebodyrescueplan.com/meditation-audio-request/

and put in the code **TBRMP1**.

Scan Me!

Using a QR code reader, you will be taken straight to the link above!

CHAPTER 2

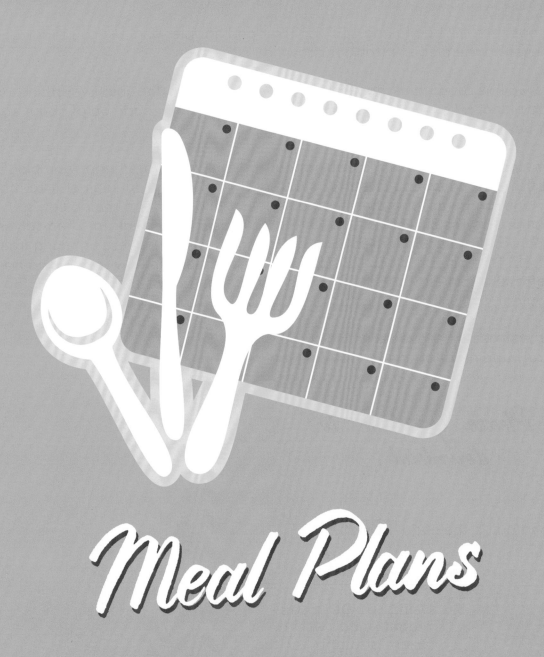

Meal Plans

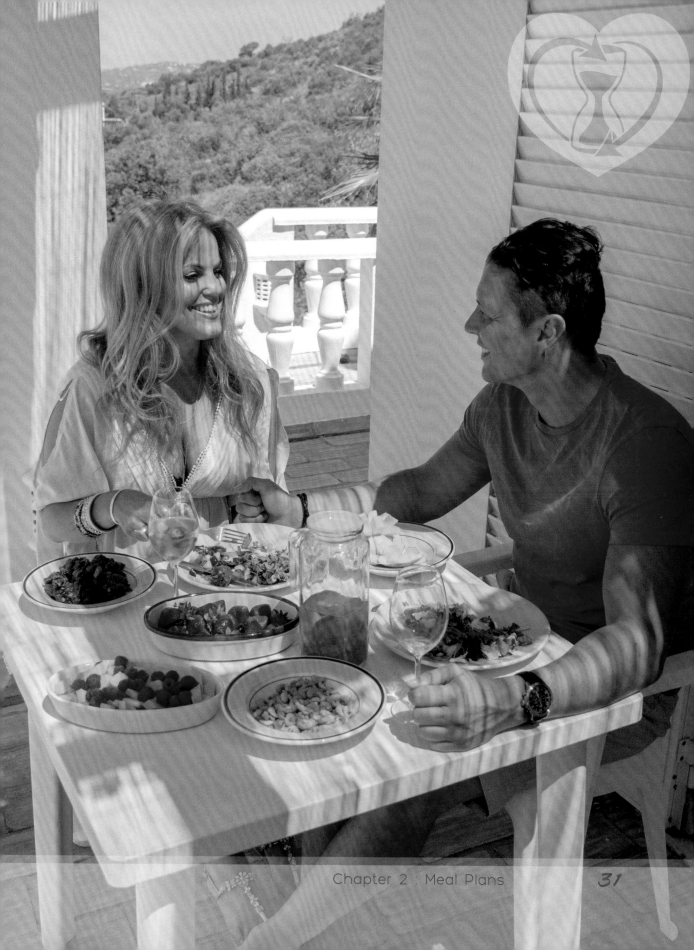

MEAL PLANS
Summer

Week 1	Breakfast	Snack	Lunch	Snack	Supper
Monday	Quinoa Apple Porridge	Tzatziki & Crudités	Pepper and Paprika Soup	Tomato & Beetroot Juice	Pasta Prawn Salad
Tuesday	Poached Eggs & Portobello Mushrooms	Apple and Greens with Lime Juice	Aubergine, Tomato & Goat's Cheese Grills with Salad	Banana & Sultana Oat Cookies	Courgette Burgers
Wednesday	High Protein Pancakes	Detox Energy Bars	Spicy Mackerel with Green Salad	Crispy Quinoa Cakes	Spicy Bean Burgers with Salad
Thursday	Mango Smoothie	Cherry Tomato & Feta Bites	Carrot and Coriander Soup	Fig Yogurt	Fishcakes with Sweet Potato
Friday	Fruity Yogurt Shake	Sweet Potato Crisps	Smoked Salmon Roll-ups	Baked Bananas with Maple Syrup & Greek Yogurt	Rice, Lentil & Beetroot Salad with Goat's Cheese
Saturday	Grapes & Yogurt	Romaine Parcels	Smoked Tofu Stir Fry	Sweet Potato Cakes	Stuffed Peppers with Salad
Sunday	Homemade Muesli	Lemon, Orange, Carrot, Apple & Spinach Juice	Rice Free Vegetable Sushi	Vegan Strawberry Ice Cream	Butternut Squash & Couscous Salad

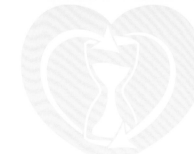

Week 2	*Breakfast*	*Snack*	*Lunch*	*Snack*	*Supper*
Monday	Carrot, Apple & Citrus Smoothie	Oaty Balls	Quinoa Salad	Raspberry Fool	Halibut and Fennel Salad
Tuesday	Puffed Rice & Yogurt with Fruit, Nuts & Seeds	Piquant Peppers with Soft Cheese & Dill	Cauliflower Soup	Açai & Maca Libido Bars	Chickpeas, Cherry Tomatoes & Rocket
Wednesday	Scrambled Egg on Toasted Rye Bread	Beetroot Chips with Curried Yogurt	Cream of Celery Soup	Sweet Potato Brownies	Tuna & Mango Salsa
Thursday	Raisin & Banana Porridge	Kale Crisps	Avocado Prawn Salad	Detox Energy Bars	Ratatouille
Friday	Stuffed Portobello Mushrooms	Rice Cakes & Avocado	Tomato & Mushroom Omelette	Butter Bean, Tomato & Basil Spread	Cauliflower Pizza
Saturday	Buckwheat Porridge	Sweet Potato Crisps	Goat's Cheese on Toast & Walnut Salad	Vegan Rice Pudding	Lentil Burgers with Salad
Sunday	Fruity Omelette	Chocolate Smoothie	Veggie Burgers & Sweet Potato Chips	Frozen Mango & Vanilla Yogurt	Jacket Potato & Salad

Week 3	Breakfast	Snack	Lunch	Snack	Supper
Monday	Mango Smoothie	Avocado & Tomato on Rye Bread	Pepper & Paprika Soup	Stuffed Baked Apples	Baked Sweet Potato & Salad
Tuesday	Fruit Kebabs	Coconut Oil Popcorn	Red Salad	Romaine Parcels	Quinoa Falafels & Tahini Sauce
Wednesday	Poached Eggs & Portobello Mushrooms	Acai & Maca Libido Bars	Salmon Steaks & Green Salad	Tomato & Beetroot Juice	Jacket Potato & Salad
Thursday	Strawberry & Banana Shake	Plantain Chips	Carrot & Leek Soup	Coconut Rice Squares	Pasta Prawn Salad
Friday	Apple & Ginger Porridge	Cherry Tomato & Feta Bites	Carrot & Coriander Soup	Vegan Strawberry Ice Cream	Spicy Vegetable Stew
Saturday	Fruity Yogurt Shake	Piquant Peppers with Soft Cheese & Dill	Traffic Light Stir Fry	Vegan Rice Pudding	Fishcakes with Sweet Potato
Sunday	Lemon, Orange, Carrot, Apple & Spinach Juice	Red Bean Dip	Asparagus Salad Topped with Poached Eggs	Crispy Quinoa Cakes	Rice, Lentil & Beetroot Salad with Goat's Cheese

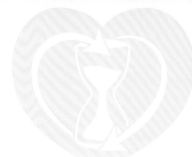

Week 4	Breakfast	Snack	Lunch	Snack	Supper
Monday	Homemade Muesli	Raspberry Fool	Tomato Soup	Tzatziki & Crudités	Tuna & Mango Salsa
Tuesday	Scrambled Egg on Toasted Rye Bread	Fig Yogurt	Spicy Mackerel with Green Salad	Kale Crisps	Courgette Burgers
Wednesday	Quinoa Apple Porridge	Oaty Balls	Goat's Cheese on Toast & Walnut Salad	Beetroot Chips with Curried Yogurt	Stuffed Peppers with Salad
Thursday	High Protein Pancakes	Chocolate Smoothie	Quinoa Salad	Avocado & Tomato on Rye Bread	Summer Veg Gratin
Friday	Buckwheat Porridge	Apple & Greens with Lime Juice	Smoked Tofu Stir Fry	Banana & Sultana Oat Cookies	Spicy Bean Burgers with Salad
Saturday	Stuffed Portobello Mushrooms	Avocado Toast	Asparagus & Pear Salad with Almonds	Banana & Date Squares	Spicy Baked Chickpea Salad
Sunday	Grapes and Yogurt	Coconut & Sultana Cookies	Rice Free Vegetable Sushi	Sweet Potato Brownies	Cauliflower Pizza

Week 1	Breakfast	Snack	Lunch	Snack	Supper
Monday	Tomato & Mushroom Omelette	Lemon, Orange, Carrot, Apple & Spinach Juice	Smoked Tofu Stir Fry	Coconut Rice Squares	Courgette Burgers
Tuesday	Raisin & Banana Porridge	Red Bean Dip	Celeriac Salad	Sweet Potato Crisps	Butternut Squash & Tomato Salsa with Salad
Wednesday	Quinoa Apple Porridge	Kale Crisps	Jacket Potato & Salad	Detox Energy Bars	Cauliflower Pizza
Thursday	Eggs on Top	Avocado Toast	Pepper & Paprika Soup	Beetroot Chips with Curried Yogurt	Veggie Burgers & Sweet Potato Chips
Friday	Stuffed Portobello Mushrooms	Plantain Chips	Traffic Light Stir Fry	Vegan Rice Pudding	Spicy Vegetable Stew
Saturday	Homemade Muesli	Romaine Parcels	Cream of Celery Soup	Fig Yogurt	Sweet Potato, Lentil & Coconut Curry
Sunday	Scrambled Egg on Toasted Rye Bread	Sweet Potato Cakes	Spicy Baked Chickpea Salad	Crispy Quinoa Cakes	Ratatouille

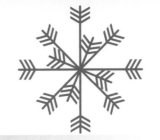
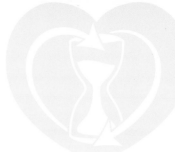

Week 2	Breakfast	Snack	Lunch	Snack	Supper
Monday	High Protein Pancakes	Sweet Potato Brownies	Roasted Red Pepper Soup	Tomato & Beetroot Juice	Penne Pasta Bake
Tuesday	Fruity Omelette	Oaty Balls	Carrot & Leek Soup	Kale Crisps	Filled Potato Shells & Salad
Wednesday	Apple & Ginger Porridge	Açai & Maca Libido Bars	Quinoa Falafels & Tahini Sauce	Banana & Date Squares	Lentil Burgers with Salad
Thursday	Poached Eggs & Portobello Mushrooms	Banana & Sultana Oat Cookies	Tomato Soup	Cauli & Courgette Cookies with Sweet Potato Topping	Thai Coconut Curry
Friday	Puffed Rice & Yogurt with Fruit, Nuts & Seeds	Avocado & Tomato on Rye Bread	Tuna & Mango Salsa	Baked Bananas with Maple Syrup & Greek Yogurt	Spicy Bean Burgers with Salad
Saturday	Kedgeree	Plantain Chips	Pepper & Paprika Soup	Coconut & Sultana Cookies	Butternut Squash & Couscous Salad
Sunday	Eggs on Top	Chocolate Smoothie	Aubergine, Tomato & Goat's Cheese Grills with Salad	Tomato & Beetroot Juice	Fish Curry

Week 3	Breakfast	Snack	Lunch	Snack	Supper
Monday	Stuffed Portobello Mushrooms	Fig Yogurt	Goat's Cheese on Toast & Walnut Salad	Sweet Potato Cakes	Baked Sweet Potato & Salad
Tuesday	High Protein Pancakes	Detox Energy Bars	Pasta Prawn Salad	Lemon, Orange, Carrot, Apple & Spinach Juice	Ratatouille
Wednesday	Homemade Muesli	Plantain Chips	Cauliflower Soup	Crispy Quinoa Cakes	Smoked Tofu Stir Fry
Thursday	Buckwheat Porridge	Stuffed Baked Apples	Salmon Steaks & Green Salad	Beetroot Chips with Curried Yogurt	Spicy Rice with Vegetables
Friday	Tomato & Mushroom Omelette	Avocado Toast	Carrot & Coriander Soup	Red Bean Dip	Fishcakes with Sweet Potato
Saturday	Scrambled Egg on Toasted Rye Bread	Kale Crisps	Halibut & Fennel Salad	Oaty Balls	Veggie Burgers & Sweet Potato Chips
Sunday	Fruity Omelette	Coconut & Sultana Cookies	Beetroot Soup	Vegan Rice Pudding	Fish Stew

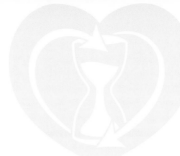

Week 4	Breakfast	Snack	Lunch	Snack	Supper
Monday	Homemade Muesli	Apple & Greens with Lime Juice	Tomato Soup	Coconut Oil Popcorn	Butternut Squash & Tomato Salsa with Salad
Tuesday	Poached Eggs & Portobello Mushrooms	Romaine Parcels	Carrot, Parsnip & Onion Soup	Açai & Maca Libido Bars	Mixed Vegetable Curry
Wednesday	Apple & Ginger Porridge	Crispy Quinoa Cakes	Traffic Light Stir Fry	Banana & Sultana Oat Cookies	Tomato & Tofu Casserole
Thursday	Quinoa Apple Porridge	Chocolate Smoothie	Pumpkin Soup	Sweet Potato Crisps	Rice & Veg with Beans
Friday	High Protein Pancakes	Avocado & Tomato on Rye Bread	Tuna & Mango Salsa	Vegan Rice Pudding	Stuffed Peppers with Salad
Saturday	Raisin & Banana Porridge	Detox Energy Bars	Coconut & Prawn Soup	Tomato & Sweet Potato Brownies	Vegetable Korma
Sunday	Kedgeree	Banana & Date Squares	Asparagus Salad Topped with Poached Eggs	Beetroot Juice	Three Bean Casserole

MEAL PLANS
Vegetarian

Week 1	Breakfast	Snack	Lunch	Snack	Supper
Monday	Mango Smoothie	Oaty Balls	Pepper & Paprika Soup	Tomato & Beetroot Juice	Traffic Light Stir Fry
Tuesday	High Protein Pancakes	Açai & Maca Libido Bars	Tomato & Mushroom Omelette	Raspberry Fool	Sweet Potato, Lentil & Coconut Curry
Wednesday	Puffed Rice & Yogurt with Fruit, Nuts and Seeds	Piquant Peppers with Soft Cheese & Dill	Spicy Baked Chickpea Salad	Plantain Chips	Ratatouille
Thursday	Apple & Greens with Lime Juice	Sweet Potato Cakes	Cream of Celery Soup	Coconut Rice Squares	Stuffed Peppers with Salad
Friday	Raisin & Banana Porridge	Chocolate Smoothie	Beetroot Soup	Tzatziki & Crudités	Spicy Vegetable Stew
Saturday	Poached Eggs & Portobello Mushrooms	Avocado Toast	Veggie Burgers & Sweet Potato Chips	Cherry Tomato & Feta Bites	Butternut Squash & Couscous Salad
Sunday	Grapes & Yogurt	Rice Cakes, Eggs & Cukes	Carrot, Parsnip & Onion Soup	Vegan Strawberry Ice Cream	Lentil & Beetroot Salad with Goat's Cheese

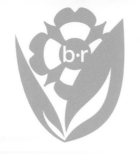
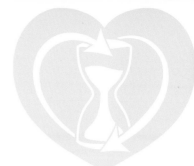

Week 2	Breakfast	Snack	Lunch	Snack	Supper
Monday	Quinoa Apple Porridge	Sweet Potato Crisps	Courgette Burgers	Beetroot Chips with Curried Yogurt	Vegetable Korma
Tuesday	Stuffed Portobello Mushrooms	Cauli & Courgette Cookies with Sweet Potato Topping	Tomato Soup	Açai & Maca Libido Bars	Quinoa Falafels & Tahini Sauce
Wednesday	Fruity Yogurt Shake	Red Bean Dip	Jacket Potato & Salad	Raspberry Fool	Cauliflower Pizza
Thursday	Eggs on Top	Banana & Sultana Oat Cookies	Carrot & Leek Soup	Carrot, Apple & Citrus Smoothie	Spicy Rice with Vegetables
Friday	Fruit Kebabs	Fig Yogurt	Goat's Cheese on Toast & Walnut Salad	Banana & Date Squares	Baked Sweet Potato & Salad
Saturday	Homemade Muesli	Romaine Parcels	Asparagus Salad Topped with Poached Eggs	Sweet Potato Crisps	Butternut Squash & Tomato Salsa with Salad
Sunday	Scrambled Egg on Toasted Rye Bread	Detox Energy Bars	Lentil Burgers with Salad	Coconut Oil Popcorn	Mixed Vegetable Curry

Week 3	Breakfast	Snack	Lunch	Snack	Supper
Monday	Apple & Greens with Lime Juice	Sweet Potato Brownies	Quinoa Salad	Avocado & Tomato on Rye Bread	Pumpkin Soup
Tuesday	Grapes & Yogurt	Coconut & Sultana Cookies	Carrot & Coriander Soup	Frozen Mango & Vanilla Yogurt	Rice & Veg with Beans
Wednesday	Fruity Omelette	Detox Energy Bars	Rice Free Vegetable Sushi	Vegan Strawberry Ice Cream	Vegetable Korma
Thursday	Buckwheat Porridge	Crispy Quinoa Cakes	Cauliflower Soup	Banana & Sultana Oat Cookies	Traffic Light Stir Fry
Friday	Stuffed Portobello Mushrooms	Piquant Peppers with Soft Cheese & Dill	Bean Salad & Rocket	Cherry Tomato & Feta Bites	Rice, Lentil & Beetroot Salad with Goat's Cheese
Saturday	Eggs on Top	Oaty Balls	Summer Veg Gratin	Kale Crisps	Spicy Vegetable Stew
Sunday	Apple & Ginger Porridge	Chocolate Smoothie	Spicy Bean Burgers with Salad	Avocado & Tomato on Rye Bread	Cauliflower Pizza

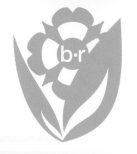
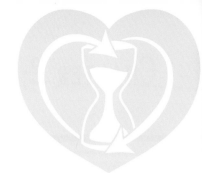

Week 4	Breakfast	Snack	Lunch	Snack	Supper
Monday	Lemon, Orange, Carrot, Apple & Spinach Juice	Vegan Rice Pudding	Quinoa Falafels and Tahini Sauce	Fruity Yogurt Shake	Baked Sweet Potato and Salad
Tuesday	Baked Sweet Potato & Salad	Kale Crisps	Asparagus & Pear Salad with Almonds	Tzatziki & Crudités	Spicy Rice with Vegetables
Wednesday	Homemade Muesli	Fig Yogurt	Goat's Cheese on Toast & Walnut Salad	Tomato & Beetroot Juice	Ratatouille
Thursday	Scrambled Egg on Toasted Rye Bread	Crispy Quinoa Cakes	Courgette Burgers	Beetroot Chips with Curried Yogurt	Filled Potato Shells & Salad
Friday	Raisin & Banana Porridge	Butter Bean, Tomato & Basil Spread	Aubergine, Tomato & Goat's Cheese Grills with Salad	Baked Bananas with Maple Syrup & Greek Yogurt	Stuffed Peppers with Salad
Saturday	Fruity Omelette	Coconut & Sultana Cookies	Roasted Red Pepper Soup	Plantain Chips	Thai Coconut Curry
Sunday	Poached Eggs and Portobello Mushrooms	Avocado Toast	Smoked Tofu Stir Fry	Vegan Rice Pudding	Butternut Squash & Couscous Salad

MEAL PLANS
Gluten Free

Week 1	Breakfast	Snack	Lunch	Snack	Supper
Monday	Raisin & Banana Porridge	Lemon, Orange, Carrot, Apple & Spinach Juice	Tomato & Mushroom Omelette	Plantain Chips	Quinoa Salad
Tuesday	Buckwheat Porridge	Chocolate Smoothie	Cream of Celery Soup	Tzatziki & Crudités	Mixed Vegetable Curry
Wednesday	Stuffed Portobello Mushrooms	Cherry Tomato & Feta Bites	Coconut & Prawn Soup	Banana & Sultana Oat Cookies	Ratatouille
Thursday	Grapes & Yogurt	Apple & Greens with Lime Juice	Chickpeas, Cherry Tomatoes & Rocket	Sweet Potato Brownies	Pumpkin Soup
Friday	Homemade Muesli	Beetroot Chips with Curried Yogurt	Asparagus Salad Topped with Poached Eggs	Vegan Rice Pudding	Courgette Burgers
Saturday	Kedgeree	Fruity Yogurt Shake	Celeriac Salad	Vegan Strawberry Ice Cream	Cauliflower Pizza
Sunday	Eggs on Top	Oaty Balls	Smoked Tofu Stir Fry	Fig Yogurt	Stuffed Peppers with Salad

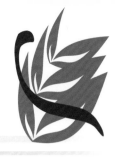
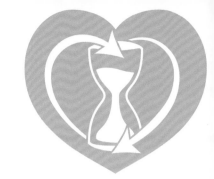

Week 2	Breakfast	Snack	Lunch	Snack	Supper
Monday	Poached Eggs & Portobello Mushrooms	Sweet Potato Crisps	Carrot & Leek Soup	Frozen Mango & Vanilla Yogurt	Filled Potato Shells & Salad
Tuesday	Carrot, Apple & Citrus Smoothie	Romaine Parcels	Roasted Red Pepper Soup	Coconut Rice Squares	Spicy Vegetable Stew
Wednesday	Apple & Ginger Porridge	Sweet Potato Cakes	Tuna & Mango Salsa	Tomato & Beetroot Juice	Lentil Burgers with Salad
Thursday	Fruity Omelette	Raspberry Fool	Bean Salad & Rocket	Vegan Rice Pudding	Tomato & Tofu Casserole
Friday	Homemade Muesli	Açai & Maca Libido Bars	Carrot, Parsnip & Onion Soup	Stuffed Baked Apples	Baked Sweet Potato & Salad
Saturday	Grapes & Yogurt	Red Bean Dip	Traffic Light Stir Fry	Plantain Chips	Sweet Potato, Lentil & Coconut Curry
Sunday	Mango Smoothie	Piquant Peppers with Soft Cheese & Dill	Halibut & Fennel Salad	Coconut & Sultana Cookies	Summer Veg Gratin

Week 3	*Breakfast*	*Snack*	*Lunch*	*Snack*	*Supper*
Monday	Quinoa Apple Porridge	Oaty Balls	Smoked Salmon Roll-ups	Tzatziki & Crudités	Butternut Squash & Tomato Salsa with Salad
Tuesday	Fruity Yogurt Shake	Sweet Potato Cakes	Tomato Soup	Coconut Rice Squares	Fish Stew
Wednesday	Buckwheat Porridge	Kale Crisps	Aubergine, Tomato & Goat's Cheese Grills with Salad	Detox Energy Bars	Spicy Rice with Vegetables
Thursday	Homemade Muesli	Beetroot Chips with Curried Yogurt	Avocado Prawn Salad	Açai & Maca Libido Bars	Baked Sweet Potato & Salad
Friday	Carrot, Apple & Citrus Smoothie	Fig Yogurt	Rice Free Vegetable Sushi	Cauli & Courgette Cookies with Sweet Potato Topping	Butternut Squash & Couscous Salad
Saturday	Apple & Ginger Porridge	Crispy Quinoa Cakes	Veggie Burgers & Sweet Potato Chips	Cherry Tomato & Feta Bites	Salmon Steaks & Green Salad
Sunday	Poached Eggs & Portobello Mushrooms	Chocolate Smoothie	Pepper & Paprika Soup	Frozen Mango & Vanilla Yogurt	Thai Coconut Curry

The Body Rescue Maintenance Plan

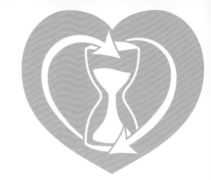

Week 4	Breakfast	Snack	Lunch	Snack	Supper
Monday	Quinoa Apple Porridge	Detox Energy Bars	Carrot & Coriander Soup	Kale Crisps	Red Salad
Tuesday	Raisin & Banana Porridge	Lemon, Orange, Carrot, Apple & Spinach Juice	Beetroot Soup	Sweet Potato Crisps	Tuna & Mango Salsa
Wednesday	Fruity Omelette	Coconut & Sultana Cookies	Cauliflower Soup	Red Bean Dip	Vegetable Korma
Thursday	Buckwheat Porridge	Sweet Potato Brownies	Asparagus & Pear Salad with Almonds	Tomato & Beetroot Juice	Fishcakes with Sweet Potato
Friday	Eggs on Top	Coconut Oil Popcorn	Spicy Mackerel with Green Salad	Baked Bananas with Maple Syrup & Greek Yogurt	Rice & Veg with Beans
Saturday	Strawberry & Banana Shake	Banana and Sultana Oat Cookies	Quinoa Falafels & Tahini Sauce	Raspberry Fool	Fish Curry
Sunday	Stuffed Portobello Mushrooms	Piquant Peppers with Soft Cheese & Dill	Rice, Lentil & Beetroot Salad with Goat's Cheese	Crispy Quinoa Cakes	Spicy Baked Chickpea Salad

CHAPTER 3

THE BODY RESCUE
Kitchen

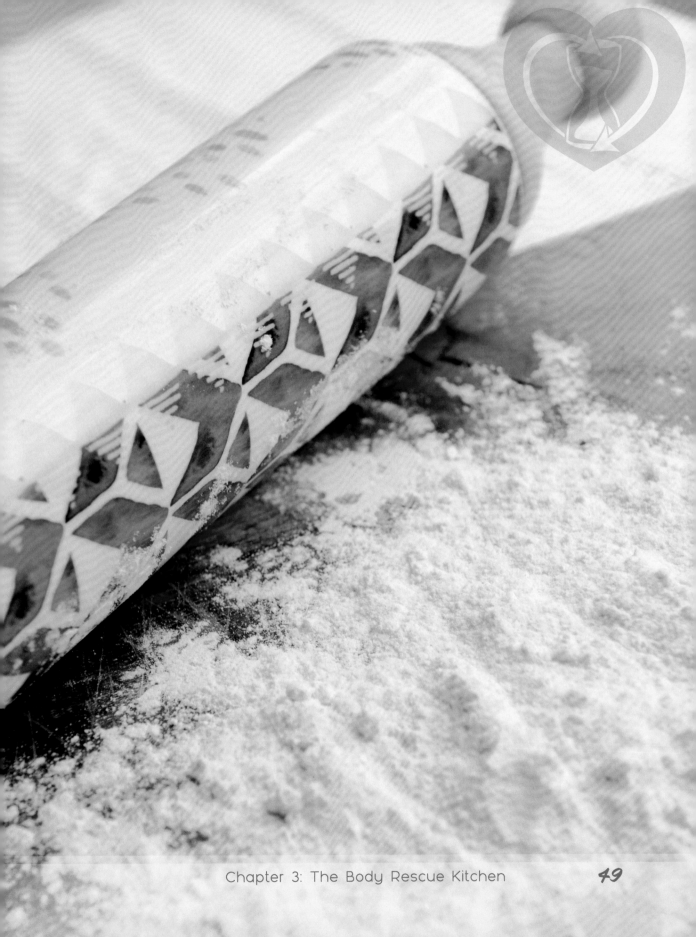

CHAPTER 3: THE BODY RESCUE Kitchen

We each see our kitchen in a different way. For some of us it's purely functional, a place where meals are made, served and eaten. For others, it's a caring and creative place, somewhere we can take time over putting together nutritious, delicious dishes to nurture ourselves and those we love. For yet others, the kitchen is the centre of the home, somewhere everyone gathers together at least once a day to share a meal and talk about what's happening in their lives.

Irrespective of how you view your kitchen it is, in a very real sense, the central source of wellness in your home. The ingredients you choose, the equipment and cooking methods you employ, the combination and portion size of the meals you prepare and serve, are all elements that can directly affect your health and your family's health, every bit as much as your attitude and commitment to exercise.

Thinking about your kitchen as a place where you can shape and improve your fitness and health is a great mindset to develop. After all, every time you prepare a meal, you make nutritional choices that directly affect well-being.

In addition, the kitchen can be a place to find true peace or pleasure, somewhere relaxing and restorative. For many of us the cosy environment, enticing smells and humble rituals of the kitchen can be wonderfully soothing. Uncomplicated, repetitive actions such as chopping vegetables, stirring a pot of food and even cleaning can be calming and satisfying, and give us a few minutes to unwind and de-stress.

As with so many things, how you feel about it will affect your experience. If you see your kitchen as a stressful place where tedious but necessary chores are carried out, then chances are it will always make you feel stressed and depressed. But it needn't take a huge change of attitude to start seeing it as a haven, a place of meditation, and the healthy heart of your warm, welcoming home.

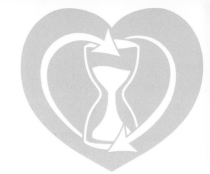

I read a wonderful mindfulness book recently which talked about doing the washing up and being mindful – the most laborious of tasks we can associate with pain and boredom. But actually when you are mindful of how amazing it is you have running water, a kitchen, soap, a warm house etc., it becomes a lot more pleasurable!

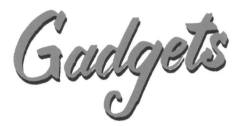

There are many kitchen gadgets available to take at least some of the grind out of some of the things we do while preparing food. While if you enjoy doing certain things, such as chopping herbs or grating vegetables, the 'hard' way, there's no need to stop, by letting technology take the strain – as we have with the use of clothes washers and dishwashers, for example – you can boost your enjoyment of cooking and free up more time to spend with the people and pastimes you love.

Juicer

Juicers are far more commonplace now and there are many more to choose from than was the case even just five years ago; juicing has really proved its worth! While you can process some fruits and vegetables in a blender or food processor, if you are going to juice hard, dense fruits and vegetables, like apples and carrots, you really need a dedicated juicer.

There are three main types, those being: masticating juicers, which knead and grind the raw material against a screen to extract the juice; centrifugal juicers, which work at high speed and contain a blade that chops the items into small pieces, then uses centrifugal force to separate the juice from the pulp; and triturating juicers, top of the line machines that can deal with pretty much anything you care to throw at them.

The best thing to do is to set a budget and conduct some research to see which is the best juicer for you, as some of these machines represent a substantial investment. As well as bearing in mind how much they cost, you might want to take into account how much space they'll take up in your kitchen! They can also make a noise, too – one of my lovely clients, Lindsay, bought a blender and a soundproof box, as she lives in a flat in London and didn't want to upset her neighbours – how courteous!

Blender / hand blender

Also known as a liquidiser, these are used to mix and puree foods. Among other things, they are great for soups and smoothies, and the more heavy duty machines can also chop ice.

A blender might be a stand-alone machine or an attachment you fit on to a food processor. A hand blender – or stick blender – is smaller and is generally used for smaller amounts of food or liquid, or in instances when you want to take the blender to the pan or bowl rather than tipping liquids into a separate container.

Food processor

Food processors first appeared on the market back in the 1940s and while they've come a long way since then, they still perform the same basic functions.

A food processor can save you a lot of time when it comes to slicing, grating, chipping or chopping fruits, vegetables, and cheese (for example) as well as mixing batters and doughs in a fraction of the time it can take to do it by hand.

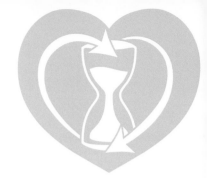

There is a wide range of machines available, ranging in price from a few pounds to several hundred, so do your research and get the one that best suits your needs.

Mini chopper

When it comes to chopping small quantities of things, such as herbs, for example, a mini chopper is very useful and can save you a lot of time. I have a great little hand chopper that I especially like using for chopping onions and garlic, as that way I don't get tears and my hands don't smell.

With prices starting at just a few pounds, they can be a worthwhile addition to your kitchen.

Slow cooker

While slow cookers – or crockpots – were first used in the early 1970s, there has been a steady rise in their popularity in recent years as more and more people have realised they are both a great way to cook delicious, nutritious meals, and also a wonderfully efficient use of time. With so many of us 'time poor' these days, that alone is a tremendous attraction.

The principle of slow cooking is simple – the contents of the ceramic pot are slowly cooked in whatever liquid you choose to use at a temperature usually just below boiling point. Because of the low-power heating element, there isn't a fast, vigorous boil; instead your food cooks gradually over several hours. This makes slow cookers ideal for stews, casseroles, soups, hotpots, and some curry recipes.

Cooking food for a long time usually results in the loss of a lot of nutrients, but this is less of a problem with a slow cooker. The lower temperature means fewer nutrients are destroyed by the cooking process, while the lid means any that do escape will not evaporate, but remain in the liquid.

One criticism of slow cooking is that food needs to be prepared in advance, often first thing in the morning before people head off to work, and not everyone wants to invest that amount of effort. However, the trade-off is that you can head out for the day knowing that when you get home there will be a hot, tasty meal waiting to be served up, with no other effort required. In addition, slow cookers are both inexpensive to buy and extremely energy efficient, with energy consumption only slightly higher than a domestic light bulb.

Soup maker

Soup makers might be relatively new kids on the block compared to some of the other gadgets mentioned here, but they have certainly hit the ground running. Earlier this year it was reported that sales of soup makers had overtaken sales of juicers.

If you love soup – and who doesn't? – then you'll love soup makers! You are completely in control: you decide what to put in it and what consistency of soup you want, and you can go from having a pile of raw ingredients to a bowl of fresh, hot, steaming soup in less than half an hour. And, in common with slow cookers, nutrients are retained.

There are three basic types: the hotplate, the jug and the blender, although they all essentially do the same thing: cook and puree soup.

The first type typically has a hotplate in the bottom, and you would put those ingredients that need to be sautéed in first, followed by the rest and the stock. You decide the consistency you want and, as well as cooking your soup, the machine also blends it for you.

The second type has a heating element in the base and a mixing paddle in the top, and you add all your ingredients and choose the settings for your soup.

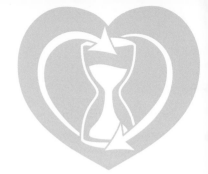

The last type is basically a blender with the ability to cook your soup.

If you like the idea of a soup maker, as always do your research. There are lots of reviews and recipes online, so check them out and see which suits you best.

Some blenders also double up as a soup maker, as they heat the vegetables as they are blending them.

Bread maker

Bread makers are useful machines – like soup makers, you measure in the raw ingredients, choose your settings, then come back to hot cooked food. A bread maker mixes, proves and bakes, and turns out a consistently good loaf every time.

The great thing about them is that you control what goes into the bread you bake. There are no issues about additives or nasties, you put in only good, healthful ingredients.

Again, there is a wide range of machines to choose from, and which you buy is likely to depend on what you need from it. More basic machines will make only a loaf of bread, but the more advanced models are also capable of making different types of bread, different sizes of loaf, cakes, and even jam and compote!

Halogen ovens

A halogen oven is a compact, stand-alone cooking unit comprising a transparent glass bowl, a lid containing the heating element, and a fan that helps circulate the heat. When the oven is switched on, the halogen lamp generates an instant and intense heat, resulting in a highly efficient oven that heats food quickly and uses much less energy than a standard oven.

Halogen ovens are surprisingly versatile; you can use them for roasting and baking, and some ovens come with accessories for cooking rice or making toast.

They also offer health benefits as they are designed to cook food evenly without the unnecessary addition of oil or fat, and their design also allows fat to drain away from food while it cooks. The fast cooking time is important – because food cooks so quickly, it retains more of the nutrients that would normally be lost during conventional cooking.

Dehydrator

You may even want to invest in a dehydrator, they're great for making dried fruit and vegetable snacks and crispbreads. They're also very healthy – as you don't heat the food up to high temperatures, you retain more nutrients.

Useful Utensils

It's not just the big things that can make life easier; there are many small utensils that can really make a difference to cooking. Again, you can do things by hand if you choose – maybe because you find it therapeutic – but if you don't want to, you don't have to. Here are just some of the ones you might find useful.

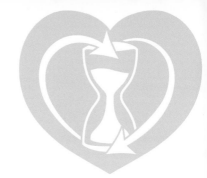

Y-shaped peeler

You can peel your vegetables with a knife if you wish, but many people find they pare away a lot of the flesh in the process, which is both wasteful and means you lose out on the nutrients just below the peel. A swivel peeler might be an improvement on a knife, but a Y-shaped peeler – with the blade sitting horizontally above the handle – is considered the best option by many. It takes off thin layers of both peel and flesh, and so can be used not just for peeling, but also for producing ribbons or thin chips of fruits and vegetables. It's fast, safe and easy to clean – and inexpensive to replace if you accidentally throw it out with the peelings!

Zester

A zester is a handy little utensil that removes the zest from citrus fruits in nice neat strands, while leaving the bitter pith behind. Yes, you can do much the same job by removing the zest with a Y-shaped peeler and then chopping it with a knife, but the shape of the fruit makes it difficult to get just the zest and not the pith, and it also takes longer.

Egg separator

There's a knack to separating the yolk from the white of an egg by passing it from half shell to half shell after it's been cracked open, and not everyone has it! While it's always prudent to separate eggs into a separate bowl, I wonder how many dishes have been spoiled by a little of the wrong part of the last egg to be added getting into them?

Luckily there's a simple, inexpensive utensil to take care of the task. Just crack the egg into it and the white will fall through while the yolk remains behind.

Knives

Good quality kitchen knives are essential. There are many opinions as to what constitutes a good knife – some chefs insist the handle should be riveted on to the blade, others that both should be formed out of the same piece of steel – so do your research and buy what suits your own personal needs and preferences. One bit of advice I would give, though, is not to skimp on the quality. Good knives can last a lifetime, so see the purchase as an investment and buy the best you can.

Knife sharpener

As well as good knives, you need an efficient sharpener. There are arguably more accidents caused by blunt knives than sharp ones, as they skid off rather than cut through the things you try to use them on. It can be as basic or as high tech as you like – there are all sorts out there: steels, stones, manual sharpeners and electric – but the difference between squashing and slicing tomatoes alone makes it a worthwhile investment!

Mandoline

Mandolines are essential for getting foods evenly sliced. The thickness of the slice is usually adjustable, and many can also be used to cut juliennes or to dice vegetables. Some have an adaptor that allows crinkle cutting – which could be very useful if you're struggling to get little ones to eat their veggies!

Make sure you get one with good safety features and take care while you use it, though – they are very sharp indeed.

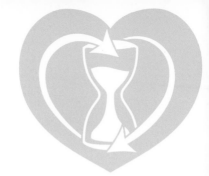

Julienne Peeler

A julienne peeler cuts vegetables into thin, even strips in a julienne cut. This is brilliant for making spaghetti shapes from vegetables like cougettes and carrots without the high carb content.

Timer

With some foods, the timing isn't important. If they stay in the oven or on the hob for an extra five or ten minutes – or even longer – it really doesn't matter. But with others, getting the timing right is essential, and you can't always use the timer on your oven. It's worth investing a few pounds in a timer for just those occasions. And it can come in handy for timing your interval training, too!

Wok

Of all the various pots, pans and dishes we use in the kitchen, the wok is perhaps the most versatile. While the most common use of a wok is in stir frying, in Asia, the wok is commonly used for a variety of cooking methods. It can be used for steaming, which is one of the healthiest cooking methods available, and you can also use a wok to smoke foods. Alternatively, you can use your wok to braise, deep fry, or even to make soup!

Non-stick woks are readily available these days, as are aluminium and steel varieties. You'll also find both flat-bottomed and round-bottomed woks available. Flat-bottomed woks are designed for modern electric cookers, while the more traditional round-bottomed wok is better suited to gas stoves. As far as size goes, generally speaking it's a case of the bigger, the better for vigorous stir frying, but take care not to buy a wok that is so large it barely fits on the hob.

CHAPTER 4

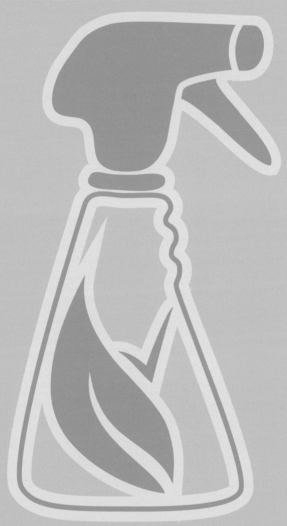

CHEMICAL FREE
Cleaning & Tips

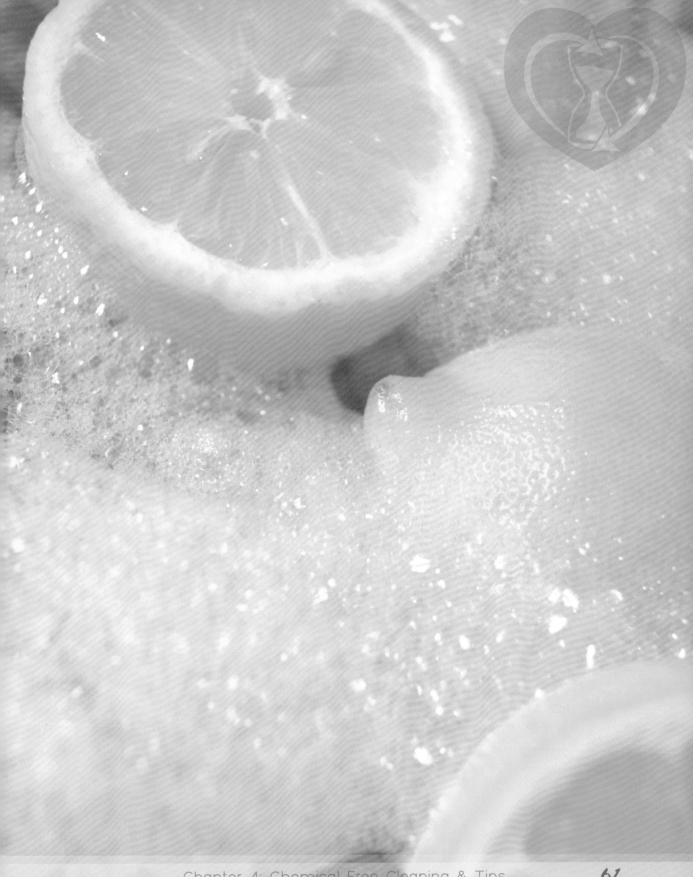

CHAPTER 4: Chemical Free
Cleaning & Tips

It's impossible to deny the huge impact human beings are having on the earth's environment and as a result many people are choosing to make lifestyle changes that will reduce their household's contribution towards polluting the planet.

When we think of environmentally toxic substances, we may look away from home and towards the big chemical corporations and the nuclear industry, but it may surprise you to know that some of the worst offenders are the enormous variety of cleaners and other chemical products found in most people's kitchens.

The majority of kitchen cleaning products use harsh chemicals to achieve results, which is how they manage to 'kill up to 99.9% of germs'. But just take a look at any average household cleaner – not even the more powerful products, like oven cleaners, and sink and drain unblockers – and you'll find the container covered in warnings telling you that you mustn't get it in your eyes or on your skin, and you must use it in a well ventilated area.

Bear in mind that any one of these products has the potential to cause dizziness, headaches or asthma attacks and then give some thought as to how it might affect the ecosystem once it's been flushed down your sink.

Many of us have been brought up to believe that 'cleanliness is next to godliness' and to associate bacteria – or germs – with dirt and disease, but there's more to it than that. Yes, some bacteria are harmful – but many aren't.

Bacteria are an essential part of the planet's ecosystem. They exist in the earth, the water and the air and they live on and in plants and animals … including us. They affect our lives and our health, and not only in detrimental ways – they inhabit our bodies and play a part in normal human physiological functions, such as digestion.

The bacteria we are exposed to can also have a direct bearing on the de-

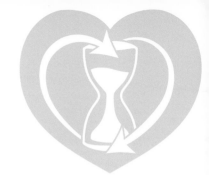

velopment of our immune systems. And that's where we hit upon a major problem.

With the use of antibacterial cleaning products, soaps and washing detergents, there's a risk of killing off the very bacteria that help develop and maintain our immune systems and other bodily functions. And in line with the concerns of the health industry that the overuse of antibiotics might actually help stronger and more virulent bugs evolve and thrive, some microbiologists are concerned that our modern over-reliance on antibacterial products may just serve to kill off weaker, 'good' bacteria ... leaving behind the stronger, more resistant and potentially more harmful strains to reproduce and thrive.

A number of studies have suggested that children raised in homes that are too clean and sterile might be more likely to suffer from allergies, asthma, and poorly-developed immune systems. According to Dr Stuart Levy, a director at Tufts University School of Medicine in Boston: 'The image that germs should be destroyed, and kids should be raised in a sterile home is a mistake. If we over-clean and sterilize, children's immune systems will not mature.'

So it seems we need to strike a balance between the need for a clean and hygienic home environment and the excessive use of specifically designed antibacterial products

An alternative approach

Making the switch from using hazardous household chemicals to adopting new green cleaning habits can take a bit of effort, but once you've taken that step, chances are you'll never look back.

There are a couple of approaches that you can take. The first is a straightforward switch from chemical products to more eco-friendly cleaners, dishwasher and laundry detergents. Most supermarkets stock environmentally friendly brands such as Ecover, Surcare and Planet Clean, and some stores also sell their own eco-friendly products. The price may be a little higher than you're used to paying, but when you take into account the fact that they're better for you and your family, as well as the environment, it's surely a worthwhile investment.

If you want to take it a step further, you can start to make your own cleaning products and solutions out of natural ingredients. I've outlined some of the basics for you here and you will find plenty more sources online, with helpful hints and tips. You may be surprised at the number of cleaning uses there are for such mundane household staples as baking soda, vinegar and lemon juice!

If you do decide to make the change from chemicals to green cleaning alternatives – and I would encourage you to give it serious consideration – there are a couple of options. Most experts suggest adopting the 'depletion' method – continue using each of your existing household products until they're finished, then choose a green replacement. Others advocate a more radical approach – once you've decided to go green, ditch all your existing chemical products and start from scratch. If you take this latter route, consider contacting your local council or recycling centre to ask if they can help you to safely get rid of your stock of hazardous household cleaning products.

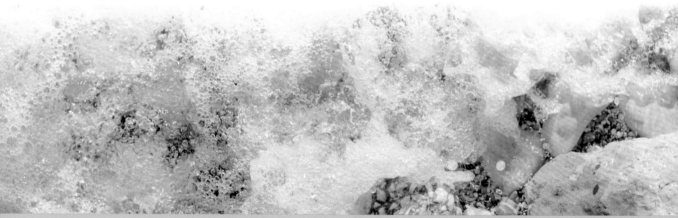

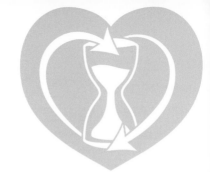

Natural Cleaning Products

Let's take a look at some of the more popular and well-established natural cleaning products we can use to keep our kitchens sparkling and hygienic ... and a couple of less well known ones that you may not be familiar with. First of all the holy trinity of all-natural kitchen cleaning products: baking soda, lemon juice, and vinegar.

Baking soda (aka bicarbonate of soda)

Baking soda is a surprisingly effective non-toxic cleaning substance that has another big advantage: it's really quite cheap, especially when bought in bulk.

You can clean kitchen surfaces by sprinkling a little baking soda onto a damp cloth and wiping down, then rinsing the surface with clean water. It's great on shiny surfaces, too; sprinkle a little on a damp cloth and wipe the mirror with it, clean with plain water, then dry off.

Baking soda also has the ability to absorb odours, so keep a pot in your fridge and sprinkle some in the kitchen bin to keep them smelling fresh.

You can even use it as a natural carpet cleaner – just sprinkle some powder onto the carpet and leave it for around fifteen minutes before vacuuming it up, leaving it clean and fresh.

Lemon juice

Lemon juice is another great all-purpose kitchen cleaner. It has strong antibacterial properties, as well as acting as a degreasing agent. An effective disinfectant and deodoriser, it also has the obvious advantage of leaving a fresh, lemony scent in your kitchen.

One way you can use it is to mix lemon juice and salt until it has a toothpaste-like consistency; this is excellent for cleaning stainless-steel sinks and fittings, and is equally effective on copper and brass – just scrub gently, then rinse with water. Combining lemon juice with baking soda and water can also work wonders on problematic spills on hob tops or oven surfaces – leave it on for fifteen minutes or so, then scrub and rinse.

Vinegar

Next on the list is good old vinegar. A fifty-fifty mixture of vinegar and water is one of the most effective surface cleaners you'll find. Put it in a spray bottle and you can use it to disinfect and deodorise kitchen tops, sinks, walls and floor – even inside the microwave. You can also clean cutlery by mixing hot water and vinegar (in a ratio of around eight parts water to one part vinegar) and letting it soak for ten minutes before rinsing and rubbing off with a cloth to remove any streaks.

Some others

While baking soda, lemon juice and vinegar may well be the holy trinity of all-natural kitchen cleaning products, there are some others that may surprise you!

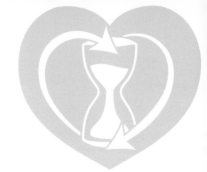

Coke

If you have any coke lying around, spare your body the last glug and use it as a useful rust cleaner. If it can remove rust, just think what it does to your insides!

Tomato ketchup

Tomato ketchup can be used to polish up tarnished metal, including brass, silverware, copper pots and pans, and stainless steel cutlery or sink surfaces. Brown sauce also works well on brass.

Black tea

If you have a hardwood floor in your kitchen, you can use black tea to clean it. Boil a pot of water on the hob, add five or six teabags and allow them to steep for ten minutes. Add some cold water to cool it down, then mop your floor as normal. It'll give it a luxurious sheen. One thing, though – this solution is for hardwood flooring, so don't use it on wood laminate flooring.

Cleaning the oven

Ovens can be horrible to clean and traditionally it's a job that requires very strong chemicals and a lot of elbow grease. However, next time you clean your oven, try the following.

Make a paste from baking soda and water and spread it on the gunk in the oven. Leave it overnight, then next day spray it with distilled vinegar and leave it for an additional hour. Finally, clean it all off with water.

Pots, pans or baking trays with burnt-on food can be cleaned by soaking them for fifteen minutes or so in hot water with baking soda added – the dirt will wipe off easily.

Descaling the kettle

Kettles need to be free of limescale to operate efficiently and also because you don't want bits of limescale in your hot drinks.

To descale, fill the kettle to just over halfway with a half and half mix of water and distilled vinegar, and allow it to boil. Once boiled, let it sit for fifteen to twenty minutes, then tip out the contents (pour through a colander lined with kitchen paper to catch all the bits) then rinse the inside thoroughly, dry it off, fill the kettle with water and boil it again. Discard at least the first fill, and if you think you can still smell vinegar, repeat the exercise.

Unblocking slow-running drains

If your sink is completely blocked, you may need to call a professional, but if it's running slow, try the following.

Put the kettle on to boil and while you're waiting, get out the baking powder and distilled vinegar.

When the kettle boils, tip the water down the plughole and follow it immediately with half a cup of baking soda. Next, mix one cup of vinegar with one cup of hot water and tip that down, too. Put the plug in and leave it for ten minutes, then boil the kettle again, take the plug out and tip a second kettle full of boiling water down. That should do the trick, and it'll work on the bathroom sink, too.

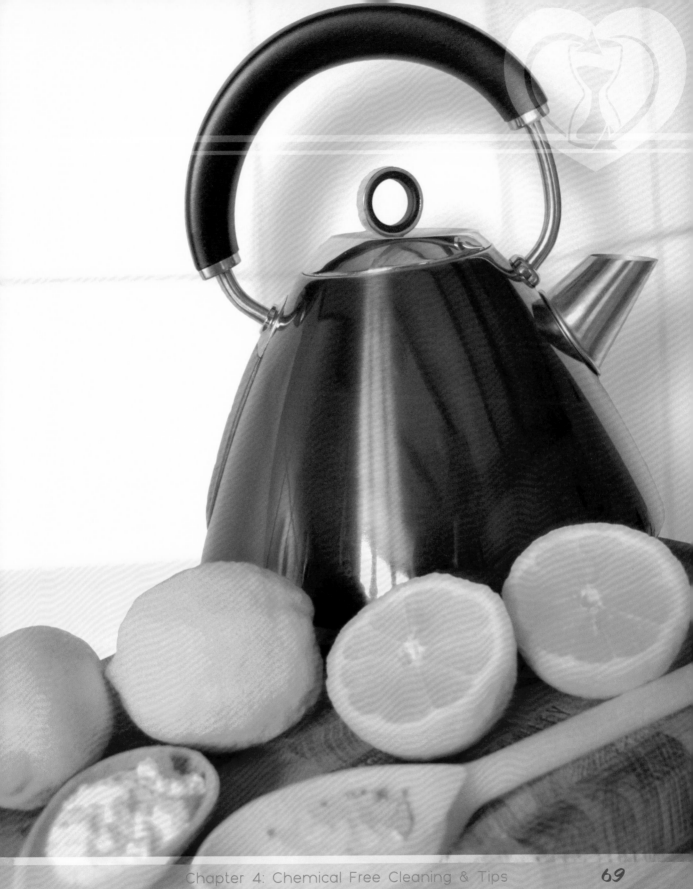

CHAPTER 5

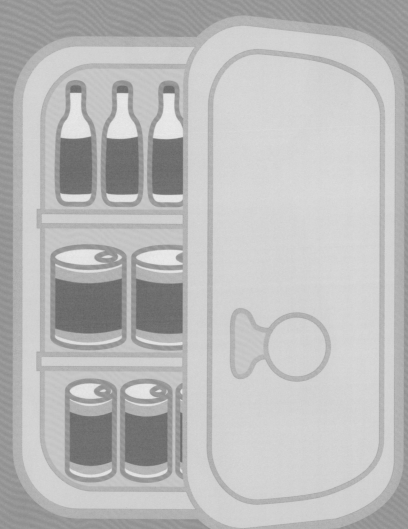

Store Cupboard
STAPLES

The Body Rescue Maintenance Plan

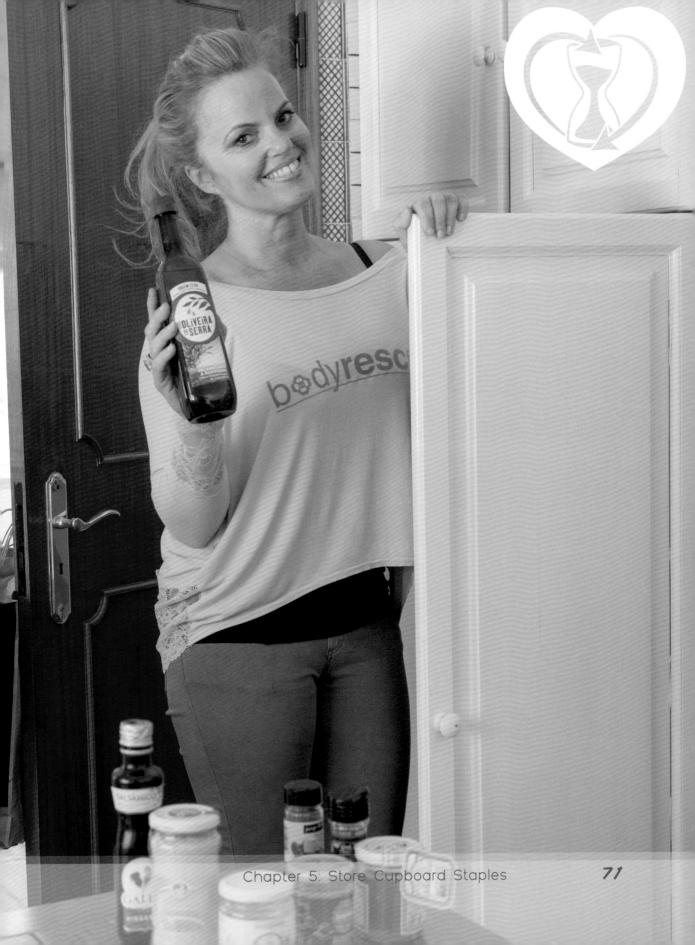

CHAPTER 5: *Store Cupboard*
STAPLES

There are certain things I think of as store cupboard staples, things I use regularly but that I don't need to buy afresh every time I need them for a recipe. These are things that come in relatively large quantities, like oils, dried or packet goods.

Below I've included a list of things that fall into this category, so you can start to build up your own store cupboard staples, too. (You don't necessarily need everything on the list – for example, you can have Himalayan salt or Celtic salt, and either honey or maple syrup. It's your choice, buy what's best for you.)

Herbs and spices

Chilli powder
Curry powder
Paprika
Smoked paprika
Cinnamon
Turmeric
Cayenne pepper
Nutmeg
Mixed spice
Ginger
Garam masala
Ground cumin
Garlic powder
Mixed dried herbs
Tarragon
Basil
Thyme
Oregano
Coriander
Marjoram
Sage
Rosemary

Oils

Olive oil
Coconut oil
Flax oil
Walnut oil

Condiments

Himalayan salt
Celtic salt
Black pepper
White pepper
Balsamic vinegar
Apple cider vinegar
Rice vinegar

Natural sweeteners

Honey
Maple syrup
Stevia
Yacon
Palm sugar
Coconut sugar

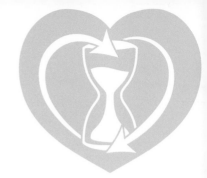

Packets and jars

Maca powder
Psyllium husk powder
Cocoa powder
Raw cacao
Porridge oats
Quinoa
Brown rice
Buckwheat
Capers
Sun-dried tomatoes
Dried apricots
Raisins
Sultanas
Dates
Wholewheat pasta
Vanilla essence

Flours

Rice flour
Almond flour
Buckwheat flour
Cornflour

Sauces

Light soy sauce
Dark soy sauce
Fish sauce

Shopping lists

I've provided some sample shopping lists for you to support the suggested meal plans, but rather than add (for example) olive oil to every list, I've included only the fresh ingredients.

Store cupboard staples are things you'll build up over time, so when you're planning to cook a recipe – or to do your weekly shop – get into the habit of first checking your store cupboard to see what things you have already and then only buy what you need – including what needs adding to or replacing in the cupboard.

Incidentally, if a recipe asks for a particular herb or spice and you realise as you're getting out your ingredients that you don't have it, don't be afraid to use substitutes. Yes, tarragon is fantastic with mushrooms and basil with tomatoes, but that doesn't mean you can't experiment a little. As a good fall back, keep some dried mixed herbs on hand.

CHAPTER 6

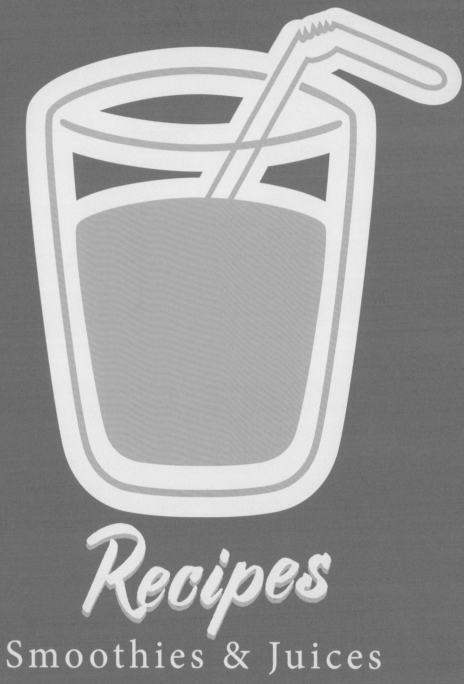

Recipes
Smoothies & Juices

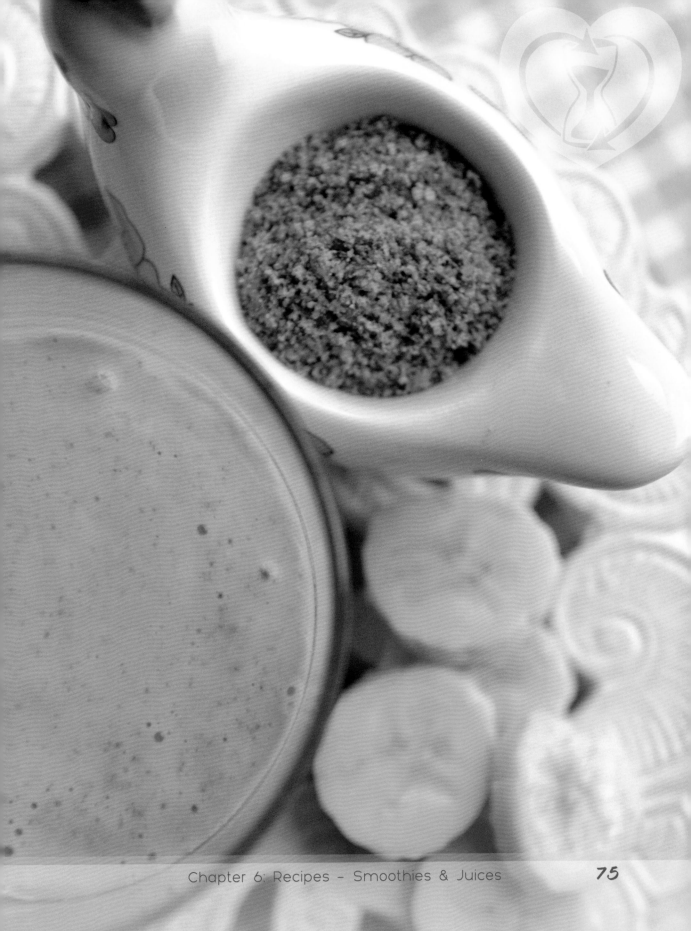

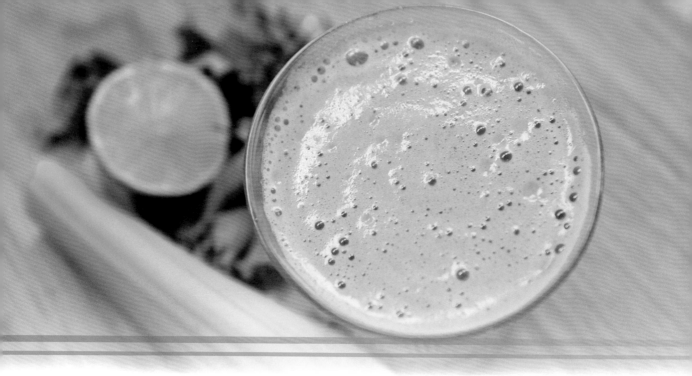

Apple & Greens with Lime Juice

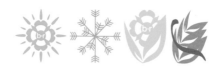

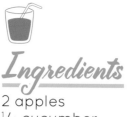

Ingredients

2 apples
¼ cucumber
1 stick of celery
1 handful of kale
1 tsp lime juice

Preparation Method

- Pass all ingredients through a juicer, stir in the lime juice, and enjoy.

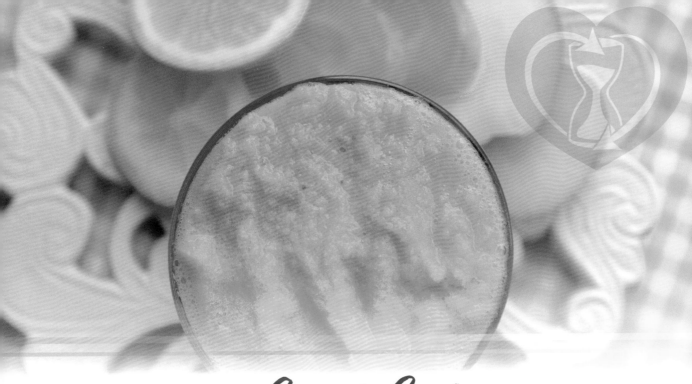

Carrot, Apple & Citrus Smoothie

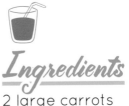

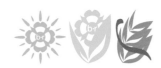

Ingredients

2 large carrots
1 apple
1 orange
1 banana

Preparation Method

• Process the carrots and apple through a juicer, and squeeze the orange.

• Put the juices in a blender with the banana and blend into a delicious smoothie

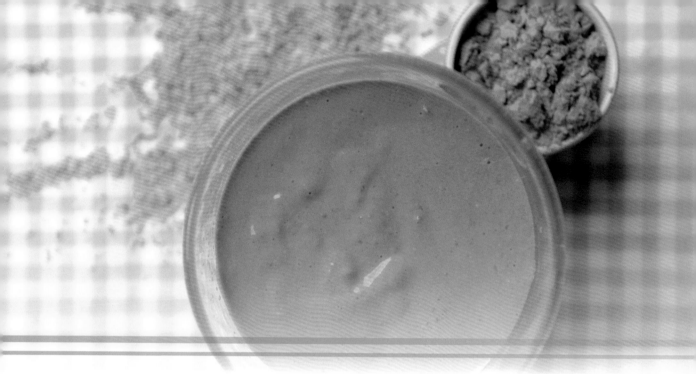

Chocolate Smoothie

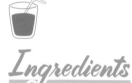

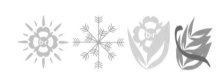

Ingredients

4fl oz / 120mls / ¹/₂ cup unsweetened almond milk, plus more to thin if desired

2 tbsps black chia seeds

3 whole Medjool dates, pitted

2¹/₂ oz / 75g / ¹/₃ cup shelled, roasted pistachios, plus more for topping

3 frozen very ripe medium bananas, peeled and sliced

2 tbsps unsweetened cocoa powder

2oz / 55g / ¹/₄ cup plain Greek yogurt (or use coconut milk yogurt for a vegan option)

1 tsp vanilla extract

Preparation Method

- Soak chia seeds in the almond milk
- Blend all ingredients together for a truly amazing drink!

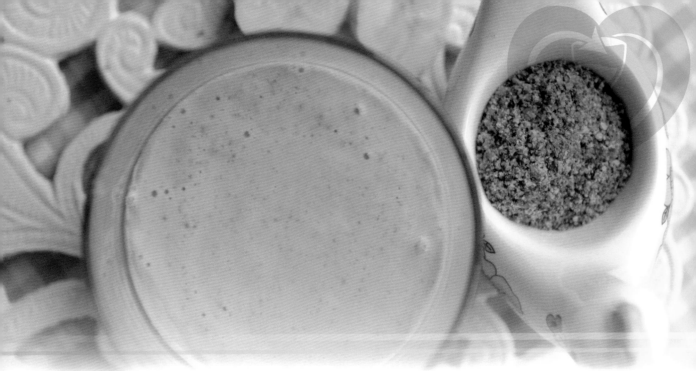

Fruity Yogurt Shake

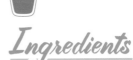

Ingredients

8oz / 225g / 1 cup (¹/₂ large pot) live yogurt
1 banana
1 tsp honey
1 tbsp milled flaxseeds

Preparation Method

• Put all the ingredients in a blender and process until smooth.

IF YOU PREFER A DIFFERENT FRUIT, USE IT INSTEAD OF THE BANANA. PEAR, MANGO AND KIWI WORK WELL IN THIS.

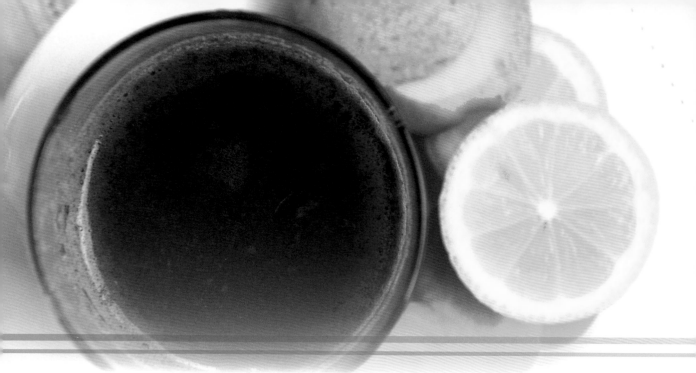

Lemon, Orange, Carrot, Apple & Spinach Juice

Ingredients

1 carrot, chopped
1 apple, cored
Handful of spinach
Juice of an orange
Juice of $\frac{1}{2}$ lemon

Preparation Method

• Pass the carrot and apple through a vegetable juicer.

• Put the vegetable juice into the blender with the other ingredients and process until smooth.

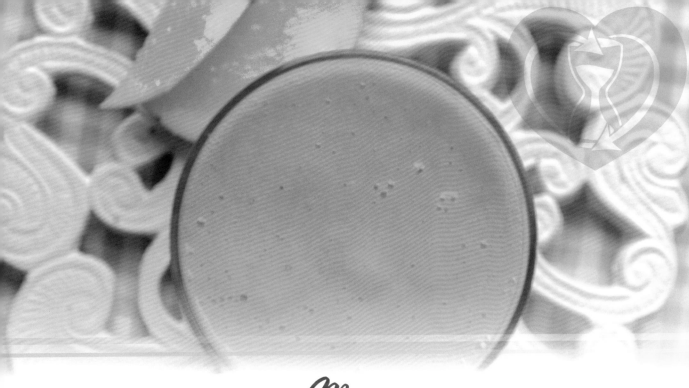

Mango Smoothie

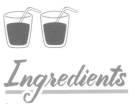

Ingredients

1 ripe mango, peeled and chopped
1 ripe banana, chopped
¼ pint / 150 mls almond milk
1 tsp honey
Few drops vanilla extract

Preparation Method

• Blend all ingredients to make a delicious, nutritious smoothie.

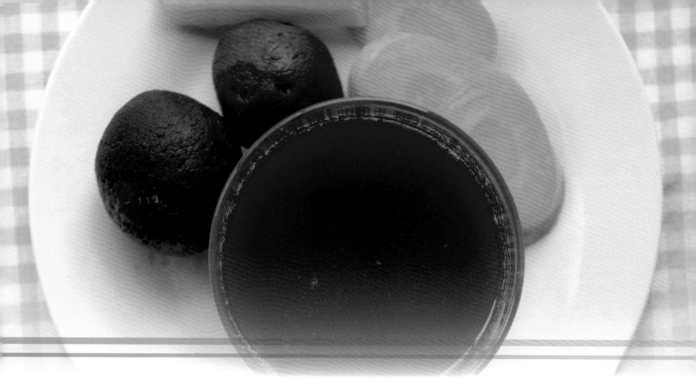

Tomato & Beetroot Juice

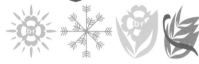

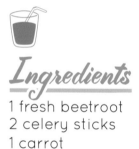

Ingredients

1 fresh beetroot
2 celery sticks
1 carrot

Preparation Method

• Put all ingredients through a juicer and drink immediately.

Beetroot contains potassium, magnesium, iron, vitamins A, B6 and C, folic acid, and antioxidants!

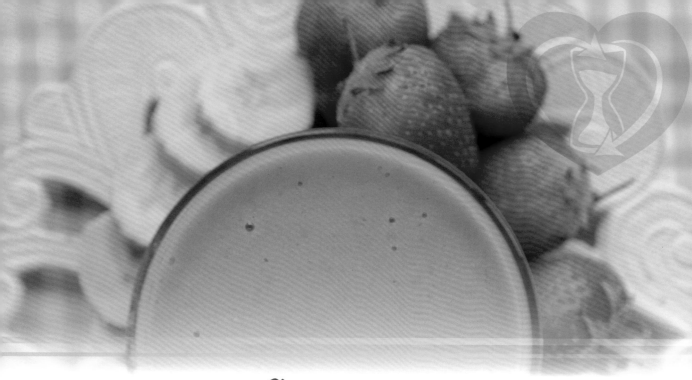

Strawberry & Banana Shake

Ingredients

8fl oz almond milk
1 frozen banana
4 large strawberries (fresh or frozen)

Preparation Method

- Place all ingredients in blender and process until thick and creamy.

Recipes

Breakfasts

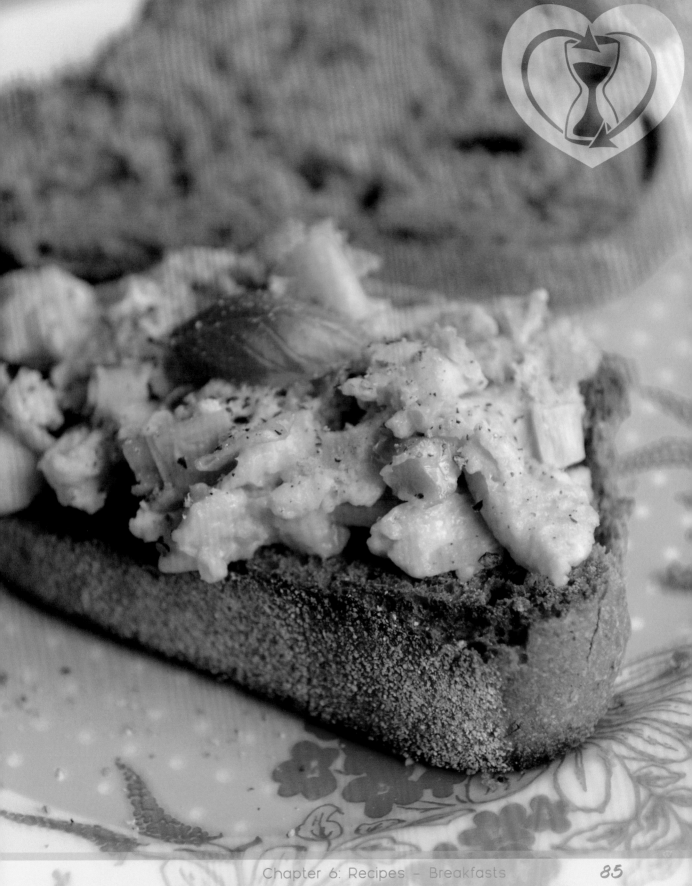

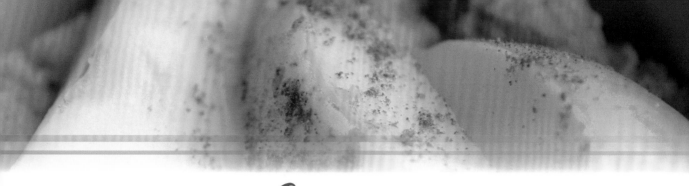

Apple & Ginger Porridge

 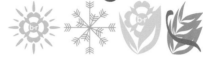

Ingredients

$2^1/_2$oz / 75g / $^3/_4$ cup porridge oats
18fl oz / 500mls / 2 cups water
1 large eating apple
Ground ginger

Preparation Method

• Cook the porridge oats in the water.

• Peel, core and chop the apple. Put in a plan with just enough water to cover and cook until soft, then drain off the water.

• Serve the porridge topped with the warm cooked apple and sprinkled with ground ginger.

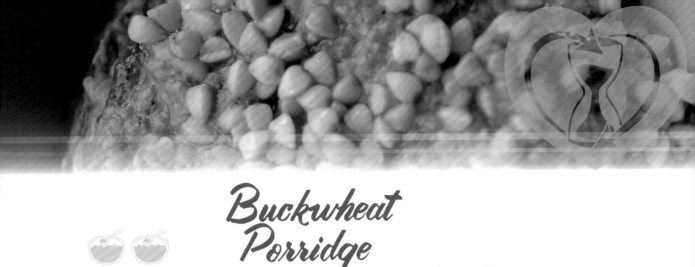

Buckwheat Porridge

Ingredients

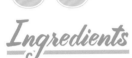

1 ripe banana
5$\frac{1}{2}$oz / 150g / $\frac{2}{3}$ cup of buckwheat soaked in $\frac{1}{2}$pint / 285mls / 1 cup of water
4oz / 115g / $\frac{1}{2}$ cup of blueberries
2$\frac{1}{2}$fl oz / 75mls / $\frac{1}{4}$ cup almond milk (any other non-dairy milk is great if you don't have almond milk)
1 tbsp almond butter
1 tbsp of chia seeds
1 tbsp of honey or maple syrup (optional)

To serve, I like some of my cinnamon pecan granola with a mixture of fresh berries, nuts, seeds, raisins, goji berries and cacao nibs.

Preparation Method

• Place the buckwheat in a bowl of water and leave overnight to soak – this is an essential step!

• Once you're ready to make your porridge, drain the water from the buckwheat and rinse it well. It will be a bit gooey, so rinse until the water coming out from your sieve is clear.

• Place two thirds of your buckwheat in a blender with the almond milk, chia seeds, banana, blueberries, almond butter and honey / maple syrup (if you're using it). Blend the mix for a minute or so until it's creamy but not totally smooth, then place it in a bowl and stir in the remaining third of the buckwheat. Serve and enjoy!

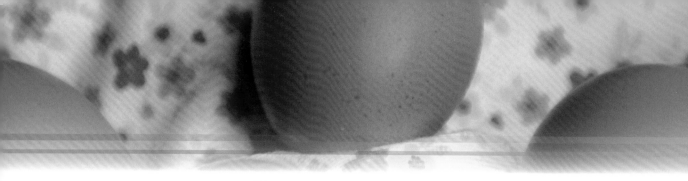

Eggs on Top

Ingredients

1 large potato, peeled and diced
2 tsps olive oil
Freshly ground black pepper
$\frac{1}{2}$ tsp chilli powder (optional)
$\frac{1}{2}$ yellow pepper, chopped
4 spring onions, chopped
4oz / 115g / $\frac{1}{2}$ cup chestnut mushrooms, sliced
2 tomatoes, diced
2 tbsps cheddar cheese, grated
2 eggs

Preparation Method

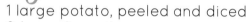

• Preheat oven to 180°C / 350°F / gas mark 4.

• In a bowl, combine a little over half the olive oil with black pepper and chilli powder, if using. Add the diced potato and mix well. Put in a baking pan and roast for 30 minutes, until browned and crispy.

• After 15 minutes or so, heat the remaining oil in a saucepan and sauté the pepper, onions, and mushrooms for 5 minutes. Add the tomato for the final minute, then set aside.

• When potatoes are done, add the sautéed vegetables to the baking pan, mix thoroughly, and return to the oven to keep warm (turn the heat right down).

• Fry or poach the eggs, whichever you prefer.

• Pile up half of the vegetable mix on each plate, sprinkle with half of the cheese, and place the eggs on top.

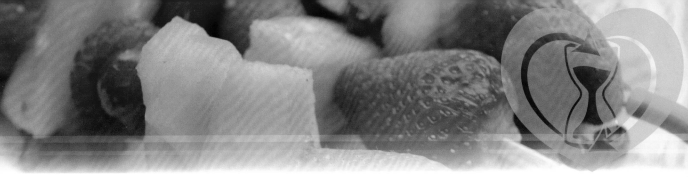

Fruity Omelette

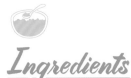

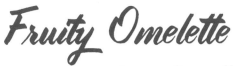

Ingredients

2 eggs
1/2 tsp cinnamon
Fistful dried fruit

Preparation Method

• Beat the eggs with the cinnamon. Heat a non-stick frying pan and pour in the egg mixture, swirling to evenly cover the base. Cook for a few minutes until set and golden underneath.

• Sprinkle the dried fruit on the top, then put under the grill for a short time to set the top.

• Fold over (or roll up) and serve.

Fruit Kebabs

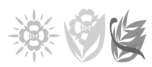

This is a great twist on a fruit salad – it's fun, healthy and great to eat!

Ingredients

A selection of your favourite fruits, cut into bite-sized pieces:
Strawberries, mango, grapes, pineapple, nectarines, apples – whatever you have available.
Honey for drizzling

Preparation Method

• Thread the fruits / chunks onto bamboo skewers. If you wish, drizzle with honey to serve.

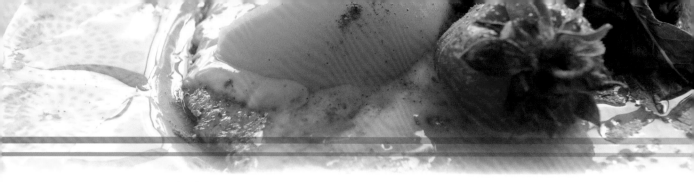

High Protein Pancakes

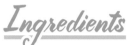

MAKES 4 PANCAKES

Ingredients

8¹/₂oz / 240g ground almonds
1 tbsp milled flaxseeds
1 tsp baking soda.
1 large egg
2oz / 60g unsweetened almond milk
8¹/₂oz / 240g coconut milk
2 tbsps coconut oil, melted

Preparation Method

• Mix the ground almonds, flaxseeds, and baking soda.

• In a separate bowl, whisk the eggs, then add the milk and oil and whisk together.

• Whisk the mixtures together gradually, adding more milk if needed, one tablespoon at a time, to make a nice pancake batter.

• Lightly oil a frying pan and heat over medium heat, and pour a cup of batter into it.

• Cook for three minutes each side.

• Serve with fruit, maple syrup, Greek yogurt etc.

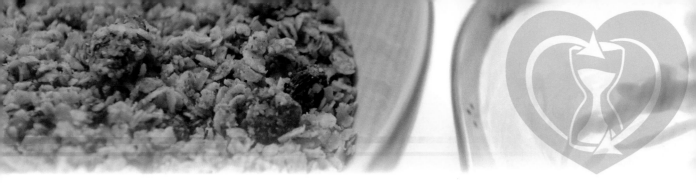

Homemade Muesli

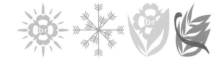

Ingredients

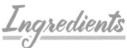

4¹/₂oz / 128g / 1¹/₂ cups oats
3¹/₂oz / 90g / ¹/₂ cup chopped dates
3¹/₂oz / 90g / ¹/₂ cup chopped walnuts and pecans
1¹/₂oz / 40g / ¹/₃ cup milled flaxseeds
1¹/₂oz / 40g / ¹/₃ cup sunflower seeds
2¹/₂oz / 75g / ¹/₃ cup raisins
2 tbsp coconut oil

TO SERVE:
Plain yogurt or fromage frais

Preparation method

- Melt the coconut oil in a wok or frying pan.
- Place all the ingredients into the pan and cook, stirring continually, for 6 minutes.
- Store your muesli in an airtight container.
- Serve a handful on some plain yogurt or fromage frais.

Milled flaxseeds are high in omega 3, which has been proven to help you lose weight.

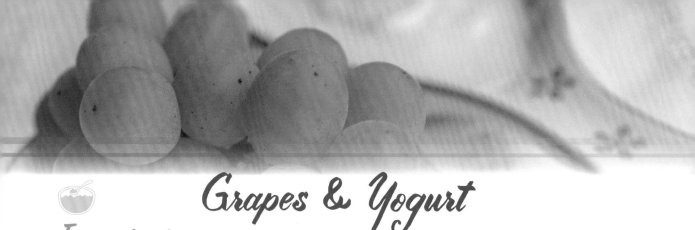

Grapes & Yogurt

Ingredients

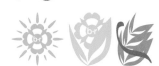

4oz / 115g / ½ cup seedless grapes
(a mix of red and green is nice)
Natural yogurt
Maple syrup
Flaxseeds

Preparation Method

• Half the grapes and put in a bowl.

• Spoon over the yogurt, drizzle with maple syrup and sprinkle with flaxseeds.

Poached Eggs & Portobello Mushrooms

Ingredients

4 eggs
4 portobello mushrooms, stems removed and wiped
Salt and freshly ground black pepper

Preparation Method

• Preheat the oven to 200°C / 390°F / gas mark 6 and line a baking sheet with baking paper.

• Place the mushrooms, gills side up, onto the paper. Bake for around 20 minutes, until tender. They may release water as they cook, so if necessary pat with kitchen paper before you put them on the plate.

• Poach the eggs, timing them to be ready at the same time as the mushrooms. Serve the mushrooms with the eggs inside, seasoned with salt and pepper.

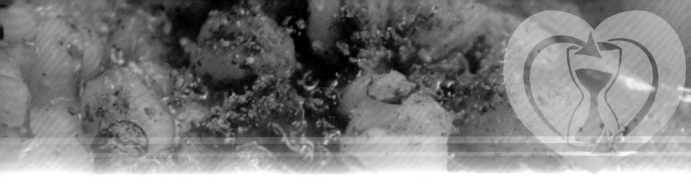

Quinoa Apple Porridge

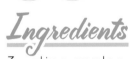

Ingredients

3 eating apples
8oz / 225g / 1 cup uncooked quinoa, soaked in water overnight
1 tsp ground mixed spice
2 tbsps honey

Preparation Method

• Peel, core and chop the apples. Put them in a saucepan with enough water to just cover them, Bring to the boil then simmer for about 15 minutes, or until tender. Drain, then mash, or puree with a hand blender.

• Drain the quinoa and put it in a saucepan with $^3/_4$ pint / 415mls / 1 $^3/_4$ cups water. Bring the mixture to a boil, then cover and lower the heat. Allow to cook for 15 minutes, or until all of the liquid has been absorbed.

• Stir in the pureed apple, mixed spice and honey, and serve.

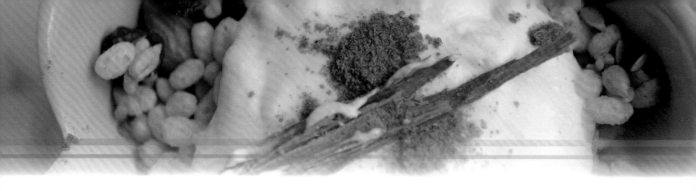

Puffed Rice & Yogurt

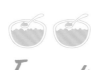

Ingredients

1 serving puffed brown rice
Nuts, seeds and dried fruit from your allowance
1 small pot natural yogurt
Cinnamon

Preparation Method

• Add the cereal, nuts, seeds and dried fruit to a bowl, top with yogurt and dust with cinnamon.

Raisin & Banana Porridge

Ingredients

1 tbsp raisins
1 frozen banana
$2^{1}/_{2}$oz / 75g / $^{3}/_{4}$ cup porridge oats
18fl oz / 500mls / 2 cups water
Cinnamon

Preparation Method

• Cook the porridge oats in the water.

• Chop the banana in a food processor and stir it and the raisins into the porridge.

• Serve sprinkled with cinnamon.

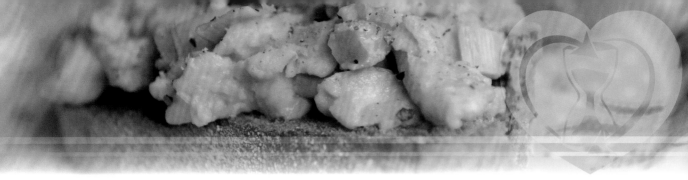

Scrambled Egg on Toasted Rye Bread

Ingredients

1 egg
1 slice rye bread
Salt and pepper
$\frac{1}{2}$ spring onion, finely chopped

Preparation Method

• Crack the egg into a non-stick pan on a medium heat. Add salt and pepper, and the chopped spring onion. At the same time, put the rye bread on to toast.

• When the egg has started to set slightly, stir it with a wooden spoon to mix it thoroughly and incorporate all the ingredients. Continue stirring until the egg is cooked; it should be just set.

• Serve the scrambled egg on the rye toast.

Cooking the egg this way means you get an attractive mix of yellow and white in your scrambled egg.

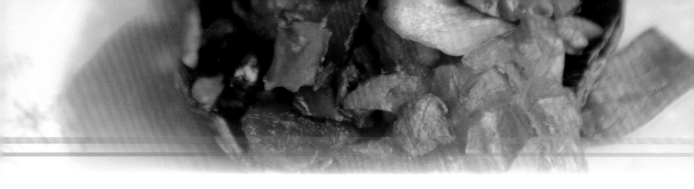

Stuffed Portobello Mushrooms

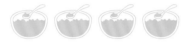

Ingredients

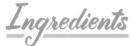

1 red onion, chopped
2 cloves garlic, crushed
8 cherry tomatoes
8 olives, sliced
4 large portobello mushrooms, stems removed and chopped

Preparation Method

• Dry fry the onion in a non-stick pan until it begins to soften. Add the garlic, tomatoes and chopped mushroom stems and cook for another 2-3 minutes. Add the olives and stir into the mix.

• Preheat the oven to 200°C / 390°F / gas mark 6 and cover a baking tray with parchment paper.

• Put the mushrooms, gills side up, on the tray and divide the cooked vegetables between them.

• Bake in the oven for 10-12 minutes, until the mushrooms are cooked.

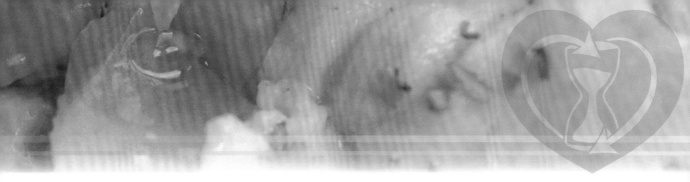

Tomato & Mushroom Omelette

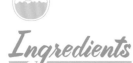

Ingredients

1 tsp coconut oil
2 eggs
2 chestnut mushrooms, sliced
4 cherry tomatoes, sliced
$1/2$ tsp dried mixed herbs
Salt and freshly ground black pepper

FOR THE SALAD:
Rocket
Tomatoes
Spring onions
Radish
Pepper

Preparation Method

• Beat the eggs and season with basil, salt and pepper.

• Heat the olive oil in a frying pan and sauté the mushrooms for 2-3 minutes. Add the eggs to the pan and at the same time turn on the grill. Using a spatula, slightly lift around the edges to allow some of the uncooked mixture to run under the sides.

• Scatter the slices of cherry tomato evenly over the top while it is still soft. Place the pan under the hot grill to finish off.

• Serve with a fresh, crisp salad made from the ingredients listed, or those of your own choice. (Add dressing as desired.)

Chapter 6

continued!

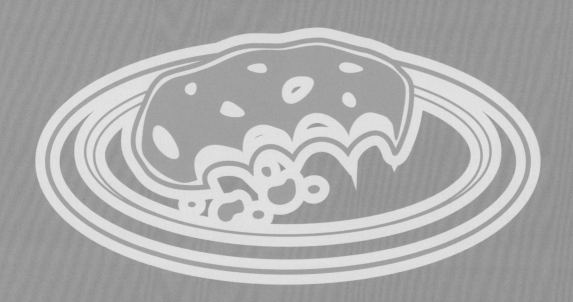

Recipes

Snacks

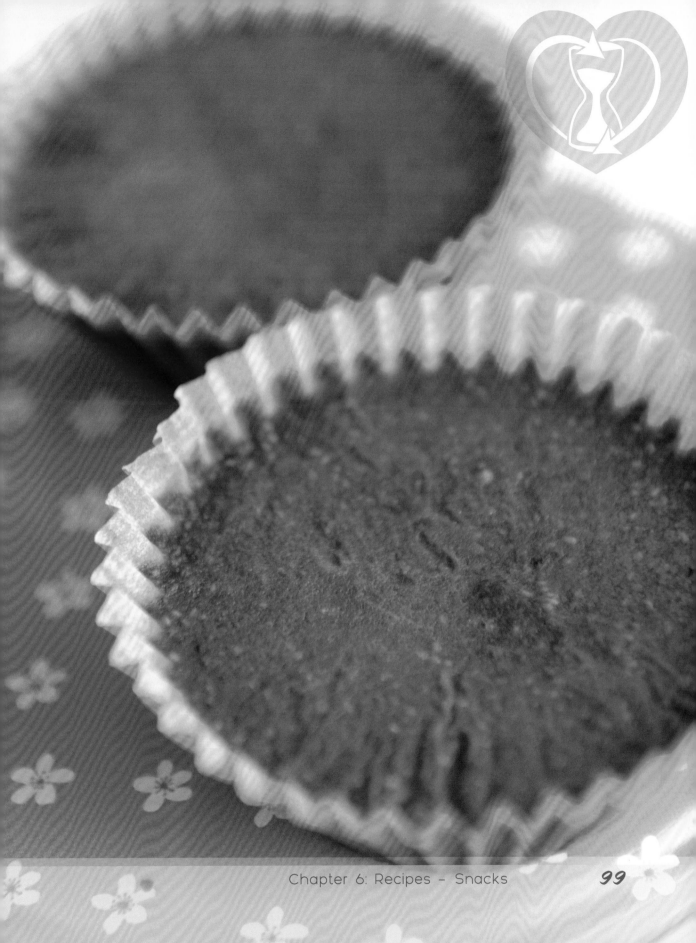

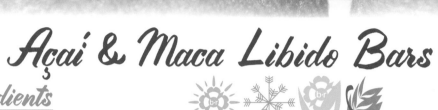

Açaí & Maca Libido Bars

Ingredients

2 tbsp Maca powder
8oz / 225g / 1 cup Açaí berries
3$\frac{1}{2}$oz / 100g / 0.4 cup almond powder
5$\frac{1}{2}$oz / 150g / $\frac{2}{3}$ cup Medjool dates (remove stones)
1 tbsp coconut oil

Preparation Method

- Blend all ingredients together.
- Roll the dough into small ball shapes.
- Place in an airtight, freezer-safe container and freeze for 30 minutes.
- All ready to eat as a delicious snack.

Maca powder is amazing for you! It's rich in B vitamins, C, and E, and has calcium, zinc, iron, magnesium, phosphorous and amino acids. Maca is widely used to raise your libido.

Avocado & Tomato on Rye Bread

Ingredients

1 slice rye bread
$\frac{1}{2}$ avocado, sliced
1 large tomato, sliced
Lime juice

Preparation Method

- Lightly toast the rye bread.
- Arrange the avocado and tomato slices on top and sprinkle with lime juice.

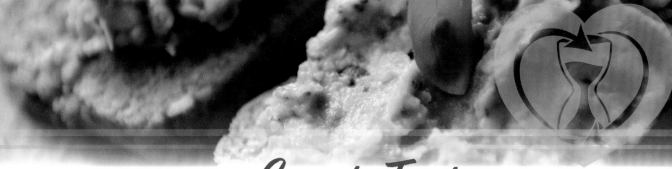

Avocado Toast

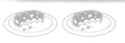

Ingredients

1 avocado
2 slices rye bread, or The Body Rescue nut bread
1 tsp lemon juice
2 tsp mixed seeds (e.g. chia, sesame, sunflower)

Preparation Method

● Toast the bread. Mash the flesh of the avocado with the lemon juice.

● Spread each slice with the avocado mixture. Sprinkle with seeds and pop back under the grill for a minute or two to heat the topping through. Serve warm.

Beetroot Chips with Curried Yogurt

Ingredients

4 beetroots
Olive oil
Salt
Dried rosemary
2 tbsps plain low-fat Greek yogurt
$1/4$ tsp curry powder

Preparation Method

● Preheat oven to 190°C / 375°F / gas mark 5.

● Thinly slice beetroots. Divide between two baking sheets and spray or very lightly drizzle with olive oil. Add a pinch of salt and the rosemary.

● Bake for 15-20 minutes or until crispy and slightly brown. Allow to cool.

● Mix together the Greek yogurt and curry powder. Serve with beetroot chips.

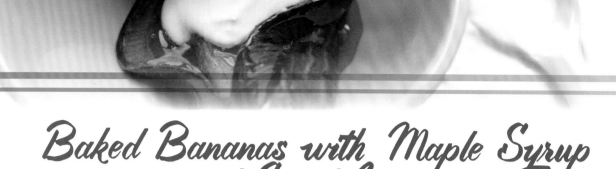

Baked Bananas with Maple Syrup and Greek Yogurt

Ingredients

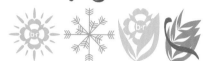

1 banana per person
Maple syrup
Greek yogurt (optional)

Preparation Method

● Preheat the oven to 200°C / 390°F / gas mark 6. Place the whole banana, in its skin, on a baking sheet. Bake for 15 minutes. (The peel will turn black.)

● Place on a plate and slit the skin carefully. Drizzle maple syrup into the hot banana. Add a dollop of Greek yogurt to the plate if you wish.

● Eat the banana from its skin with a spoon. It's delicious on its own, but the contrast with the cool, creamy yogurt, if you have it, is wonderful!

This is delicious as a breakfast, and also makes a lovely dessert. It's versatile, too. If you prefer, you can halve the bananas lengthways (still in their skin) and bake them like that, to make them easier to serve. Sprinkle with cinnamon or drizzle with syrup before you put them in the oven.

If you have a barbecue, you can wrap the bananas in foil and put them in the coals when you've finished cooking. If you make an incision in the skin, you can stuff the banana with pieces of good quality chocolate for an extra special treat.

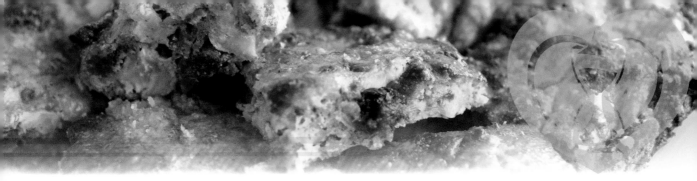

Banana & Date Squares

MAKES 20 SQUARES

Ingredients

3 large ripe bananas, mashed
8oz / 225g / 1 cup unsalted almond nut butter
3 large eggs, beaten
$^3/_4$ tsp baking soda
$^1/_4$ tsp salt
1 tsp vanilla extract
1 tsp ground mixed spice
6oz / 170g / $^3/_4$ cup chopped dates

Preparation Method

- Preheat the oven to 180°C / 350°F / gas mark 4 and line an approximately 10 inch (25cm) square baking tin with baking parchment.

- In a large bowl, mash the bananas well.

- Add the almond nut butter, beaten eggs, baking soda, salt, vanilla extract, and mixed spice, and stir well. The batter will be quite runny at this stage.

- Fold in the chopped dates, if using.

- Pour the batter into the prepared baking tin. Bake for around 30 minutes; when it's ready, the top will be browned and a skewer inserted into the middle will come out clean.

- Allow the cake to cool completely in the tin before turning out, cutting and serving. Store in an airtight container in the fridge.

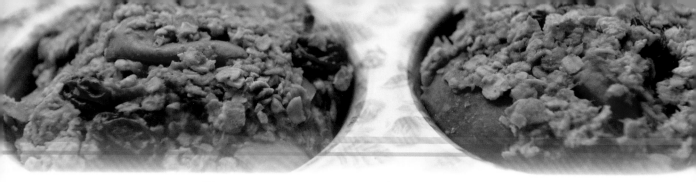

Banana & Sultana Oat Cookies

MAKES 6 COOKIES

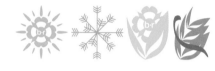

Ingredients

1 large (or 2 small) apples (e.g. Braeburn)
1 tsp lemon juice
1 tsp honey
1 large, ripe banana, mashed
4^1/$_2$oz / 128g / 1^1/$_2$ cups oats
1 tsp mixed spice
3^1/$_2$oz / 90g / ^{1}/$_2$ cup sultanas

Preparation Method

• Core, peel and chop the apples. Place in a saucepan with the lemon juice and honey and cook over a low heat until soft (5-6 minutes). Allow to cool, then mash.

• Put all of the ingredients in a bowl and mix thoroughly.

• Preheat the oven to 180°C / 350°F / gas mark 4 and line a baking sheet with baking parchment.

• Drop the mixture on to the parchment in cookie-sized portions; bake for 15-20 minutes.

This is a flexible recipe, so if you'd rather use a different fruit, such as chopped apricots, or you'd like to add some chopped nuts, go ahead. You could also use nutmeg or ginger (for example) instead of mixed spice.

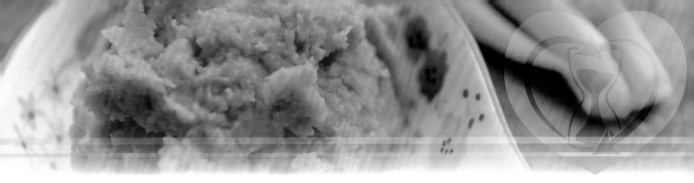

Butter Bean, Tomato & Basil Spread

Ingredients

15oz / 400g can butter beans, drained
1 tbsp tomato paste
1 clove garlic, crushed
1 tbsp lemon juice
Fresh basil (2-3 generous sprigs)
Salt and freshly ground black pepper

TO SERVE:
Celery sticks

Preparation Method

• Put all the ingredients in a blender and puree until smooth.

• Serve with celery sticks – you can either use the spread as a dip or else fill the sticks with it.

This is a tasty and versatile spread, great with crudités or spread on bread. Try it on toasted fingers of my delicious nut bread and add a salad to make a satisfying lunch!

Cauli & Courgette Cookies with Sweet Potato Topping

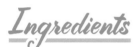

Ingredients

8oz / 225g / 1 cup courgette
4oz / 115g / $\frac{1}{2}$ cup yellow pepper
3lbs / 1.4kg / 6 cups cauliflower florets
4oz / 115g / $\frac{1}{2}$ cup of soft cheese
2oz / 60g / $\frac{1}{4}$ cup parmesan cheese, grated finely
1 egg, beaten
1 tsp of dried mixed herbs
Pinch of salt

FOR THE TOPPING:
1 large sweet potato, peeled and roughly chopped
2oz / 60g / $\frac{1}{4}$ cup plain fat free yogurt
Salt and freshly ground black pepper
Fresh coriander

Preparation Method

● To make the cookies, finely chop the vegetables using a food processor, (they should look like breadcrumbs).

● Put a small amount of water (1-2 inches) in a saucepan and bring to the boil. Add the vegetables and cook for 3-4 minutes.

● Line a colander with a tea towel and pour in the contents of the pan. Leave to go cold (or at least to cool until safe to handle) then gather up the tea

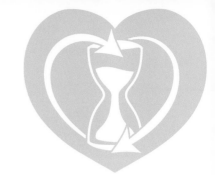

towel and squeeze out the excess water.

- Put the soft cheese, parmesan cheese, beaten egg, herbs and salt into a bowl and mix together, then add the squeezed vegetables and combine thoroughly to make a dough.

- Preheat the oven to 200°C / 390°F / gas mark 6 and line a baking tray with a baking sheet.

- Divide the dough into 8 dollops and put each one on the baking tray. Shape into rounds and flatten to about $1/4$ inch / 1cm thick (this mixture is quite soft and sticky).

- Bake for around 25 minutes until cooked through.

- Meanwhile boil or steam the sweet potato until soft (about ten minutes).

- Drain, add the yogurt, and mash until smooth. Season with salt and pepper and use to top the cookies; garnish with coriander leaves.

- Serve two per person with a crisp, healthy salad.

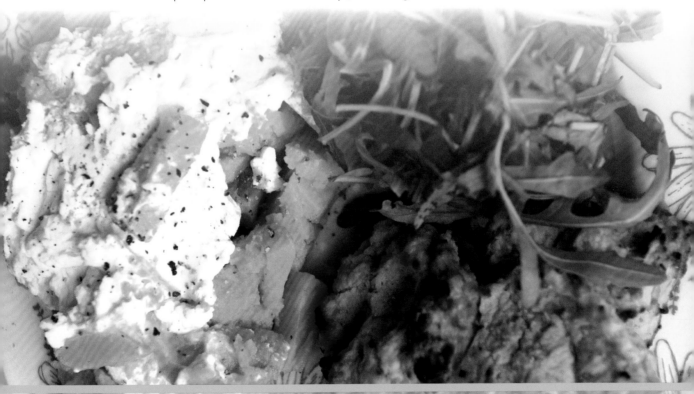

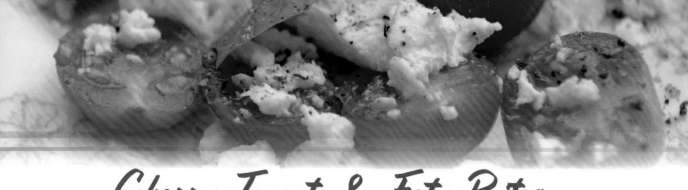

Cherry Tomato & Feta Bites

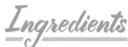

Ingredients

6 cherry tomatoes
8oz / 225g / 1 cup feta cheese
Freshly ground black pepper
6-8 basil leaves, chopped

Preparation Method

• Halve the cherry tomatoes and put 6 halves on each plate.

• Top each half tomato with crumbled feta. Season with freshly ground black pepper and sprinkle with chopped basil.

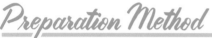

Coconut Oil Popcorn

Ingredients

4oz / 115g / $\frac{1}{2}$ cup popping porn
1 $\frac{1}{2}$ tbsps coconut oil
Himalayan salt

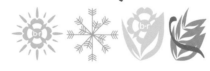

Preparation Method

• Select a large, heavy-based pan or cast-iron casserole with a lid. Melt the coconut oil over a medium heat, then add a few kernels of corn; when they pop, add the rest and put the lid on.

• Once the kernels begin popping, shake the pan every 8-10 seconds. When the popping slows right down, take the pan off the heat and shake for around 15 seconds to give the last kernels a chance to pop and prevent the ones at the bottom from burning.

• Tip into a bowl, sprinkle with the salt, and enjoy!

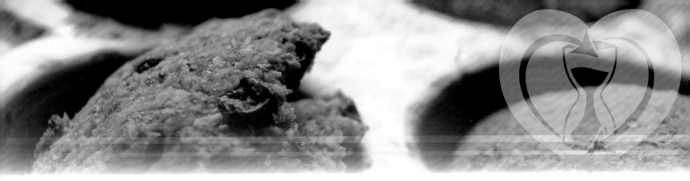

Coconut & Sultana Cookies

MAKES 12 (4 servings)

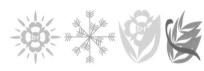

Ingredients

8oz / 225g / 1 cup almond flour
6oz / 170g / ³/₄ cup of milled flaxseeds
4oz / 115g / ¹/₂ cup desiccated coconut
2oz / 55g / ¹/₄ cup sultanas
3 egg whites
1 tsp Stevia
1 tsp lime juice
1 tbsp cornflour

Preparation Method

• Preheat the oven to 180°C / 350°F / gas mark 4 and cover a baking sheet with baking parchment.

• Combine all ingredients and mix well until they form a stiff paste.

• Divide into 12 equal portions, roll into balls then flatten to make rounds. Space out on the baking parchment.

• Bake for 12-15 minutes, then remove from the oven and cool on a rack.

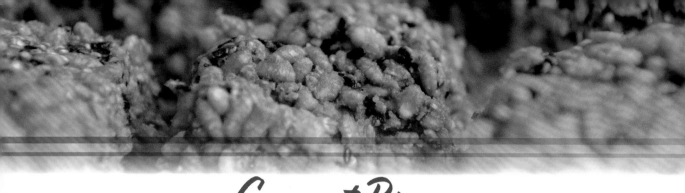

Coconut Rice Squares

MAKES AROUND 20 SQUARES

Ingredients

2^1/$_2$oz / 75g / 3 cups organic puffed rice (e.g. Kallo)
5 tbsps toasted sesame seeds
2 tbsps chia seeds
2^1/$_2$oz / 75g / ^{1}/$_3$ cup coconut oil
2^1/$_2$oz / 75g / ^{1}/$_3$ cup rice syrup
5^1/$_2$oz / 150g / ^{2}/$_3$ cup creamed coconut
Pinch of salt

Preparation Method

• Line a small baking tin (approx. 8-9 inches square) with baking paper.

• Put the puffed rice, sesame seeds and chia seeds in a large bowl.

• In a saucepan melt the coconut oil, rice syrup, and 3^1/$_2$oz / 100g / 0.4 cup of the creamed coconut and stir until melted and combined.

• Add to the rice and seeds mix and stir until well combined. Press the mix firmly into the lined tray. (Put another piece of baking paper on top so it doesn't stick to your fingers.)

• Using the same saucepan, melt the final 2oz / 55g / ^{1}/$_4$ cup of creamed coconut with the pinch of salt. Pour over the top of the mixture in the tray.

• Put the tray in the fridge until firm.

• Once it's set, slice it into small squares using a hot knife. Store in an air-tight container in the fridge.

Crispy Quinoa Cakes

MAKES 15 CAKES

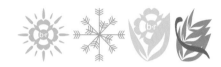

Ingredients

4 tbsps of coconut oil
1$\frac{1}{2}$ tbsps almond butter
4$\frac{1}{2}$ tbsps maple syrup
2oz / 55g / $\frac{1}{3}$ cup raw cacao powder
1$\frac{1}{2}$oz / 45g popped quinoa
Small cake cases

Preparation Method

• Put the popped quinoa into a mixing bowl and set aside.

• Place all the other ingredients in a saucepan and heat gently for a few minutes, while stirring, until the ingredients melt and combine to form a smooth mixture.

• Pour the melted mixture over the popped quinoa and stir until thoroughly combined.

• Spoon the mixture into small cake cases and place them in the freezer for around fifteen minutes or the fridge for about half an hour.

You can buy your quinoa ready popped or pop your own in a heavy bottomed pan over a medium heat. Cover with a lid and shake regularly to prevent sticking.

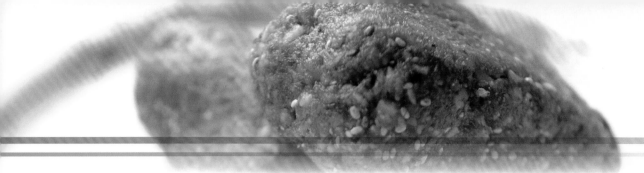

Detox Energy Bars

Ingredients

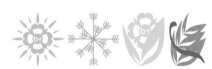

4oz / 115g / ½ cup almond
4oz / 115g / ½ cup dates
1 tsp maca powder
1 tbsp chia seeds
4oz / 115g / ½ cup dried apricots
4oz / 115g / ½ cup cashew nuts
8oz / 225g / 1 cup raisins
1 tsp vanilla extract
1 tsp cinnamon

Preparation Method

• Blend all ingredients in a blender.

• Take out the mixture and place on cellophane, then flatten it out.

• Place more cellophane on top and place in the freezer for 30 minutes or so.

• Take out and cut up into squares, all ready to eat!

These are yummy soft or hard. When you take the paste out of the blender it is more like fudge and when you freeze them they become more like toffee.

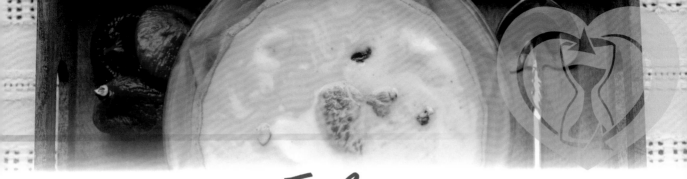

Fig Yogurt

Ingredients

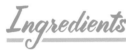
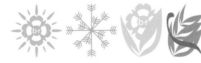

1 tbsp pine nuts, toasted
2 fresh figs
2$\frac{1}{4}$oz / 64g / $\frac{1}{4}$ cup dried figs
4$\frac{1}{2}$oz / 128g / $\frac{1}{2}$ cup plain yogurt or fromage frais
4$\frac{1}{2}$oz / 130g / $\frac{1}{2}$ cup orange juice
2$\frac{1}{4}$oz / 64g / $\frac{1}{4}$ cup raisins

Preparation Method

• Gently warm the fresh figs and raisins in a pan with the orange juice, for 2-3 minutes.

• Put the yogurt in a bowl and pour on the mixture.

• Sprinkle on the pine nuts and raisins.

Figs are a fantastic source of fibre, which helps your digestive health.
A $\frac{1}{2}$ cup serving of dried figs contains 15% of the daily adult requirement of calcium; 12% of the daily adult requirement of magnesium, 11% of potassium and 19% of iron.

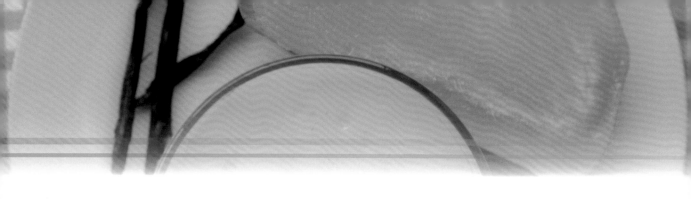

Frozen Mango & Vanilla Yogurt

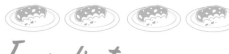

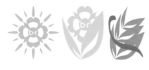

Ingredients

Flesh of 1 large mango, cubed and frozen
24fl oz / 700mls / 3 cups plain Greek-style yogurt
2 tsps vanilla extract
Juice of ½ lime
2oz / 55g / ¼ cup honey

Preparation Method

- Process all ingredients in a blender until smooth.

- Transfer into a container with a lid and freeze for 2-4 hours.

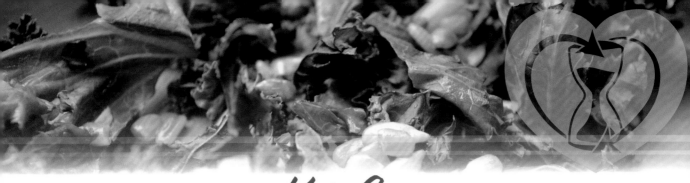

Kale Crisps

Ingredients

1 large bunch of kale
4¼oz / 120g / ½ cup sunflower seeds, finely ground
1 tbsp balsamic vinegar
1 tbsp apple cider vinegar
1 tbsp olive oil
1 tsp salt

Preparation Method

- Combine all the ingredients in a large bowl and mix into the kale.

- Heat the oven to 150°C / 300°F / gas mark 2. Place a piece of parchment paper on top of a baking sheet, then spread the kale crisps mixture evenly over the surface.

- Bake for 2 hours, keeping a close eye as it can burn easily. (You can cook the crisps quicker on a higher heat, but they retain more nutrients if you cook them more slowly.)

Kale has more calcium than milk and more iron than beef. It also is high in vitamins C, A and K, and is great for detoxing, as it's filled with fibre and sulphur.

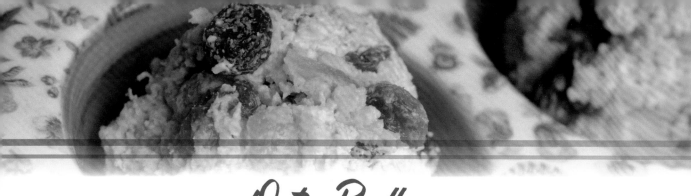

Oaty Balls

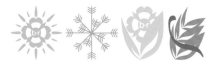

Ingredients

6oz / 170g / 2 cups oats
9oz / 250g / 1 (generous) cup dried fruit
$3^{1}/_{2}$oz / 100g / $^{1}/_{2}$ cup mixed nuts
Handful of coconut flakes
7fl oz / 200mls water mixed with yogurt
2 tbsps cashew nut butter
1 tsp cinnamon
1 tsp ground ginger

Preparation Method

• Blend together all the ingredients apart from the coconut flakes.

• Roll the mixture between your hands to form small balls. Wet the balls with the water mixture and then roll in coconut flakes.

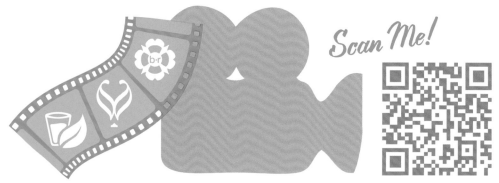

Scan Me!

I made these with my sister – you can check out our YouTube clip here:

https://www.youtube.com/watch?v= QS-LB24rILk

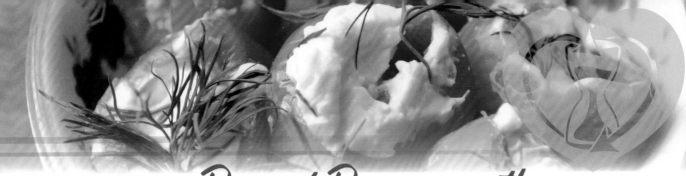

Piquant Peppers with Soft Cheese & Dill

Ingredients

Soft cheese
8 piquant red peppers (e.g. Peppadew)
Fresh dill

Preparation Method

- Remove the peppers from the jar and pat dry.
- Using a teaspoon or a piping bag, fill each pepper with soft cheese.
- Pop a sprig of dill on the cheese at the open end of the pepper.

Perfect as a snack, or serve with a crisp salad to make a satisfying lunch.

Plantain Chips

Ingredients

1fl oz / 30ml coconut oil
Coarse sea salt and ground pepper
1lb / 500g plantains or green bananas, peeled and sliced thinly on the diagonal

Preparation Method

- Preheat oven to 180°C / 350°F / gas mark 4, and line a baking sheet with parchment paper.
- Toss the plantain slices in the oil, then arrange in a single layer on the baking sheet. Season with salt and pepper.
- Bake for around 30 minutes until crisp and golden, turning the chips halfway through the cooking time.
- Drain on kitchen paper. When cooled store in an airtight container, for a couple of days

Raspberry Fool

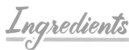

Ingredients

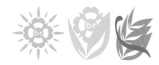

8oz / 225g / 1 cup raspberries
1 tbsp maple syrup
Zest of 1 large orange, and 1 tbsp juice
8oz / 225g / 1 cup Greek yogurt

Preparation Method

• Put the raspberries into a saucepan with the orange juice and cook on a low heat for around 5 minutes, until soft. Set aside and allow to cool, then chill in the fridge for an hour or until needed.

• Strain the raspberries, reserving the juice, and mix the fruit with the maple syrup.

• Set aside a tsp of the orange zest and mix the rest into the yogurt.

• Take two glasses and add alternate layers of fruit and yogurt. Drizzle with the reserved juice, then top with a few pieces of orange zest.

Red Bean Dip

Ingredients

1 tbsp olive oil
1 red onion, finely chopped
2 cloves garlic, crushed
Chilli powder ($1/4$ to $1/2$ tsp, as preferred)
8oz / 225g / 1 cup kidney beans
4 tbsps fromage frais
1 tsp lime juice
Salt and freshly ground black pepper
TO SERVE:
Crudités of your choice

Preparation Method

● Heat the olive oil in a frying pan and sauté the onions and garlic for 2-3 minutes. Add the chilli powder and cook for another couple of minutes.

● Allow to cool slightly, then put all the ingredients into a blender and process until smooth.

● Serve with strips of raw pepper, carrot sticks and mangetout (or other raw vegetables of your choice).

Rice Cakes & Avocado

Ingredients

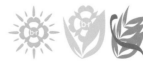

2 Biona Organic Rice Cakes with Quinoa
$1/2$ avocado, mashed

Preparation Method

● Top the rice cakes with the avocado – simple and delicious!

Rice Cakes, Eggs & Cukes

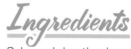

Ingredients

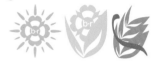

2 hard-boiled eggs
Paprika
¼ cucumber, cut into spears
2 Biona Organic Rice Cakes with Quinoa

Preparation Method

- Cut the cucumber into spears.
- Shell, and slice the eggs; place on the rice cakes and sprinkle with paprika.

Romaine Parcels

Ingredients

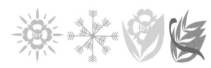

1 large avocado
1 beef tomato, chopped
½ cucumber, chopped
1 tsp lemon juice
1 head romaine lettuce

Preparation Method

- Halve the avocado, remove the stone and scoop out the flesh into a bowl. Mash the flesh thoroughly.
- Add the tomato, cucumber and lemon juice, and combine thoroughly.
- Put a spoonful of the mixture into a lettuce leaf and roll up to eat. Delicious!

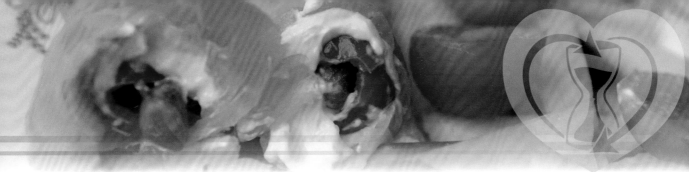

Smoked Salmon Roll-ups

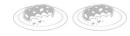

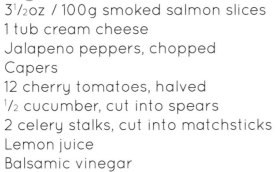

Ingredients

3$\frac{1}{2}$oz / 100g smoked salmon slices
1 tub cream cheese
Jalapeno peppers, chopped
Capers
12 cherry tomatoes, halved
$\frac{1}{2}$ cucumber, cut into spears
2 celery stalks, cut into matchsticks
Lemon juice
Balsamic vinegar
Salt and freshly ground black pepper

Preparation Method

• Separate the slices of smoked salmon and trim as necessary (or simply fold the trimmings in).

• Spread each slice with cream cheese.

• Stud the cream cheese with a mix of jalapenos and capers, then roll up the smoked salmon slices.

• Arrange on plates and add a pile each of cherry tomatoes, cucumber spears and celery matchsticks. Sprinkle the smoked salmon roll-ups with lemon juice and the cherry tomatoes with balsamic vinegar, then add salt and freshly ground black pepper to the meal to taste.

Stuffed Baked Apples

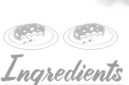

Ingredients

2 Bramley cooking apples
2 tbsps dried mixed fruit
2 tsps maple syrup
1/2 tsp grated nutmeg

Preparation Method

- Preheat the oven to 180°C / 350°F / gas mark 4.
- Core the apples, leaving around half an inch at the bottom.
- Combine all other ingredients and use to fill the apples.
- Bake the apples for 30 minutes, or until cooked (check with a skewer).

Sweet Potato Cakes

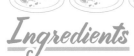

Ingredients

10 dates
2 sweet potatoes, cooked and peeled
1 tsp cinnamon
1 tsp nutmeg
1 tbsp ground almonds
1 handful of raisins
1 egg

A delicious cake to have on a detox, and nice for breakfast too!

Preparation Method

- Preheat oven to 200°C / 390°F / gas mark 6.
- Blend all of the ingredients together in a blender; mould the mixture into cake shapes and place on a brownie / cookie baking tray.
- Bake for 20-30 minutes.

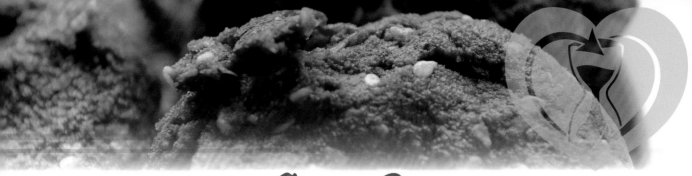

Sweet Potato Brownies

MAKES 5 BROWNIES

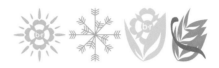

Ingredients

1 sweet potato
1 handful of sesame seeds
4oz / 120g of ground almonds
2oz / 60g of buckwheat flour
7 dates
2 tbsp raw cacao
2 tbsp honey
1 pinch of salt

Preparation Method

• Put oven on at 180°C / 350°F / gas mark 4.

• Peel and cut the sweet potatoes and cook till they are soft (steam or bake). Add the dates and sweet potato to a blender for a yummy mix. Tip into a bowl.

• Now add all the other ingredients to the bowl and mix thoroughly.

• Divide into 5 patties, place on a baking tray and cook for 20 minutes. When you take them out let them stand for at least 10 minutes to cool down or they may fall apart!

Sweet Potato Crisps

Ingredients

1 sweet potato
(approx. 9oz / 250g / 1 cup)
1 tbsp olive oil
½ tsp smoked paprika
¼ tsp paprika
Pinch of chilli powder
Pinch of Himalayan salt

Preparation Method

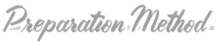

• Preheat the oven to 190°C / 375°F / gas mark 5. and cover a baking tray with parchment paper.

• Scrub the sweet potato, dry it on kitchen paper and slice it very thinly. Place the oil, smoked paprika, paprika, chilli powder and salt in a large bowl. Add the sweet potato slices and mix until evenly coated.

• Place around half the slices in a single layer on the baking sheet. Do not allow them to overlap.

• Place the sheet in the middle of the oven and bake for 10-12 minutes. (The chips are ready when the edges have curled up.)

• Slide the baking parchment from the tray onto a wire rack and let the chips cool for about 5 minutes. Meanwhile re-cover the tray with fresh baking parchment, spread out the remaining chips and cook as above.

• While the second batch are cooking, transfer the cooled chips to a serving dish. You don't need the baking tray again, so when the second batch is ready, just place the tray itself on the wire rack. (If you have two baking trays, spread each with half the chips, but bake them separately.)

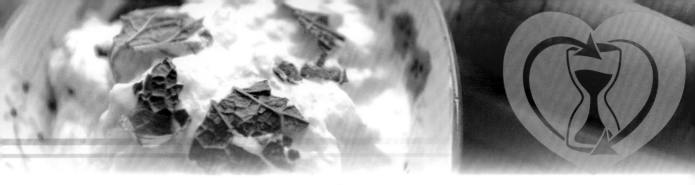

Tzatziki & Crudités

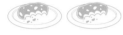

Ingredients

$^1/_2$ cucumber
1 tsp olive oil
6oz / 170g / $^3/_4$ cup Greek yoghurt
1 tsp lemon juice
1 clove of garlic, crushed
A few mint leaves, chopped

TO SERVE:
Vegetables of your choice; for example, carrot sticks, celery sticks, strips of pepper.

Preparation Method

• Peel the cucumber then cut in half lengthways and scrape out the seeds. Grate it, or chop it very finely, then squeeze it in kitchen paper or a tea towel to get some of the liquid out. Stir it into the olive oil.

• Put the yogurt in a bowl and stir through the lemon juice, garlic, and cucumber and oil mix.

• Serve in a bowl, with the crudités.

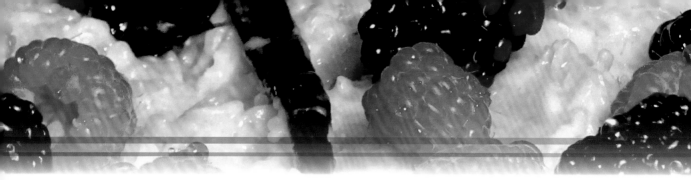

Vegan Rice Pudding

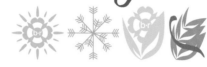

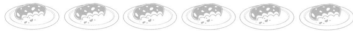

Ingredients

8oz / 225g / 1 cup Arborio rice
1 vanilla pod (split)
1 tbsp (or to taste) rice syrup, honey, or maple syrup
Pinch of salt
2.75 pints / 1.6 litres / 7 cups almond milk

TO SERVE:
Raspberries and blackberries.

Preparation Method

• Put all the ingredients apart from the milk into a saucepan.

• Cook the rice on the hob, adding the milk gradually, and stirring frequently. (It takes around 25 minutes.)

• Serve warm, with the berries on top.

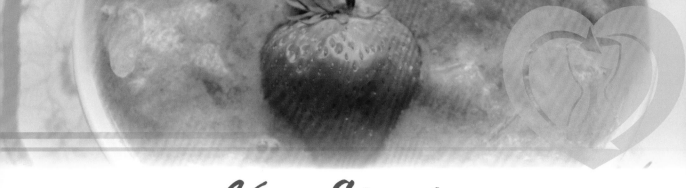

Vegan Strawberry Ice Cream

MAKES 3 PINTS / 1²/₃ LITRES

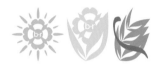

Ingredients

1¹/₂lbs / 700g / 3 cups fresh strawberries
3¹/₂oz / 100g / 0.4 cup agave nectar
²/₃ pint / 350mls rice milk
2 tsp lemon juice

Preparation Method

• Slice the berries and toss them with the agave, and let them macerate for one hour at room temperature.

• Puree the berries and their liquid in a blender with the rice milk and lemon juice.

• Chill thoroughly in a freezer.

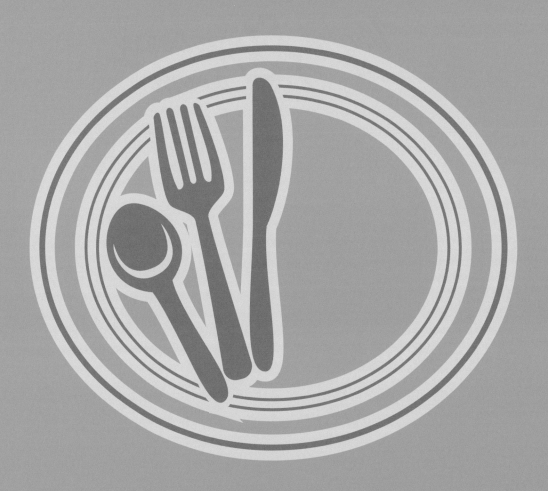

Recipes

Lunch & Supper

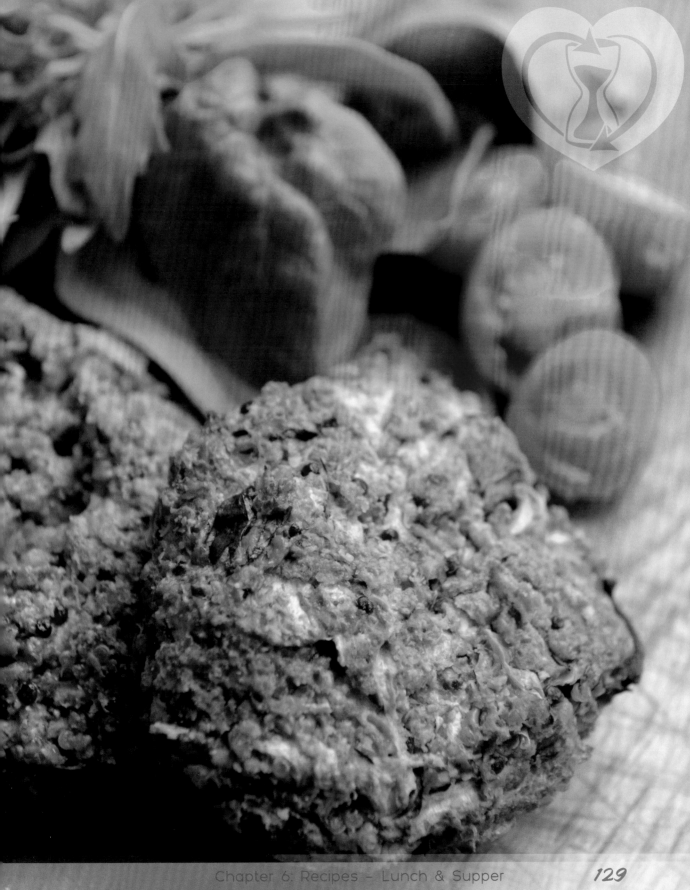

Asparagus & Pear Salad with Almonds

Ingredients

2 ripe pears
1lb / 500g / 2 cups asparagus, trimmed
1 tbsp lemon juice
2oz / 60g / $^1/_4$ cup flaked almonds
2oz / 60g / $^1/_4$ cup goat's cheese, cubed
1 head romaine lettuce (or other salad leaves)

FOR THE DRESSING:

2 tbsps olive oil
2 tbsps balsamic vinegar
1 tsp French mustard
1 tsp maple syrup
Salt and freshly ground black pepper

Preparation Method

• Trim the asparagus. Bring a pan of salted water to the boil and add the asparagus. Simmer for 7-8 minutes until tender. Drain and immediately plunge into cold water.

• Prepare the salad dressing by combining the ingredients in a bowl and whisking well to mix.

• Quarter and core the pears, then slice and add to a bowl with lemon juice. Mix well to prevent discolouration.

• Drain the asparagus and pat dry.

• Divide the romaine leaves between four plates. Arrange the asparagus and pear slices on the romaine, sprinkle with the flaked almonds and cheese and drizzle the dressing over the top.

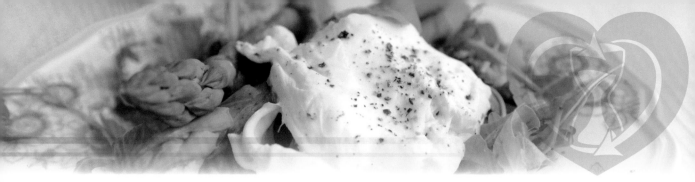

Asparagus Salad Topped with Poached Eggs

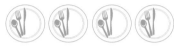

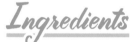

Ingredients

2 bunches asparagus, trimmed
4 large eggs
2 bags rocket

FOR THE DRESSING:
4 tbsps lemon juice
Zest of $\frac{1}{2}$ lemon
$\frac{1}{2}$ tsp garlic powder
Salt and freshly ground pepper

Preparation Method

• Steam the asparagus until tender.

• Poach the eggs, and drain.

• Meanwhile, whisk the ingredients for the dressing in a large bowl. Set aside 4 tsps.

• Toss the rocket with the dressing and divide the salad between 4 plates. Top with asparagus and a poached egg and drizzle with 1 tsp of the reserved dressing.

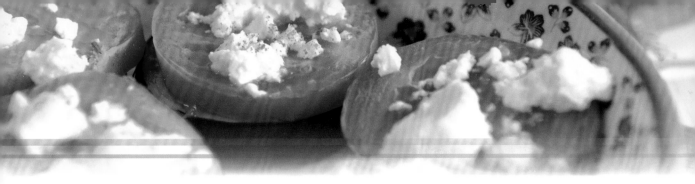

Aubergine, Tomato & Goat's Cheese Grills with Salad

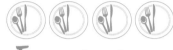

Ingredients

1 aubergine
Olive oil
4 beef tomatoes
4oz / 115g / ½ cup soft goat's cheese
Smoked paprika
FOR THE SALAD:
Rocket
Tomatoes
Spring onions
Radish
Pepper
Juice of a lemon
Salt and freshly ground black pepper

Preparation Method

• Cut the aubergine into 8 rounds, about ½ inch / 1cm thick. Brush with olive oil and grill until tender (10-15 minutes).

• Meanwhile slice the beef tomatoes. When the aubergines are ready, top each with a slice of tomato and some goat's cheese, then sprinkle with smoked paprika and place back under the grill until warmed through.

• Serve 2 per person with a fresh, crisp salad made from the ingredients listed, or those of your own choice, dressed with lemon juice and seasoned.

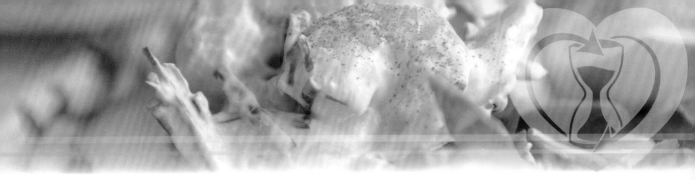

Avocado Prawn Salad

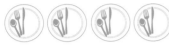

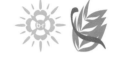

This is a new twist on an old favourite!

Ingredients

6 tbsps fromage frais
1 tbsp tomato puree
Tabasco sauce, to your taste
2 tbsps fresh chives, chopped
8oz / 225g / 1 cup cooked prawns
Salt and pepper
2 avocados, ripe and ready to eat
Paprika
Rocket
Lemon wedges

Preparation Method

• In a bowl, mix the fromage frais, tomato puree and Tabasco sauce. Stir in the chopped chives and the prawns, and season with salt and pepper.

• Halve each avocado lengthwise and remove the stone. Spoon the prawn mixture into the avocado halves, and dust with paprika.

• Place each avocado half on a bed of rocket and serve garnished with lemon wedges.

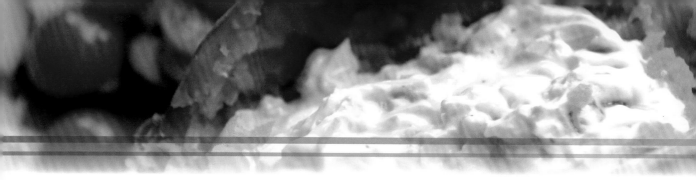

Baked Sweet Potato & Salad

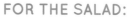

Ingredients

1 large sweet potato
2 tbsp soft cheese
1 spring onion, finely chopped
Salt and pepper

FOR THE SALAD:
Little gem lettuce
Cherry tomatoes
Cucumber
Peppers
Lemon juice

Preparation Method

• Scrub the sweet potato, prick several times with a fork, and bake in the oven at 200°C / 390°F / gas mark 6 for about an hour, or until cooked.

• Cut a cross into the potato and open up the cavity. Mix together the soft cheese and the spring onion, season with salt and pepper, and spoon into the potato. Put it back into the oven for about 5 minutes for the cheese to heat through and melt into the potato.

• Chop up the salad vegetables, mix in a bowl and dress with the lemon juice. Serve with the baked sweet potato.

The Body Rescue Maintenance Plan

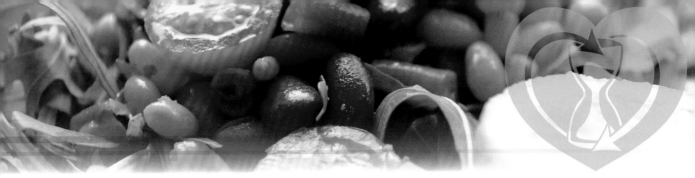

Bean Salad & Rocket

 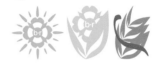

Ingredients

15oz / 400g can butter beans, drained
4oz / 115g / $\frac{1}{2}$ cup green beans
4oz / 115g / $\frac{1}{2}$ cup sweetcorn
10oz / 280g / 1 $\frac{1}{4}$ cups cherry tomatoes, halved
1 red onion, sliced thinly
1 bag rocket, washed and patted dry
1 tbsp lemon juice
2 tbsp fresh basil, chopped
Salt and freshly ground black pepper

Preparation Method

• Mix together the beans, corn, tomatoes and onion.

• Serve on a bed of rocket, dressed with lemon juice, sprinkled with basil and seasoned with salt and pepper.

If you don't like (or don't have) butter beans, substitute with another type of bean. Lima beans, cannellini beans or chickpeas would all work well in this.

Beetroot Soup

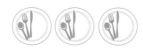

Ingredients

6 potatoes (1¼ lbs / 600g / 2½ cups)
2 beetroots (14oz / 400g / 1¾ cups)
1 tin (400ml) coconut mil
1 lemon
2 tsps of chilli flakes
2 tsps of coriander powder
1 tsp of cumin powder
2 cloves of garlic
Salt and pepper

FOR THE CROUTONS:
4 potatoes (14oz / 400g / 1¾ cups)
Salt, pepper and olive oil
1 tbsp of chilli flakes

Preparation Method

• Place the beetroots, with the skin on, onto a baking tray to roast for about an hour on 200°C / 390°F / gas mark 6.

• While these roast, peel the potatoes (just the ones for the soup) and place them into a saucepan with cold water. Bring the pan to the boil and then let them simmer for about 45 minutes, so that they're really nice and soft.

• If you want to make the potato croutons then chop the remaining potatoes (you don't need to peel these ones) into small pieces and place them on a tray with lots of olive oil plus the chilli flakes, salt and pepper. Bake for about 45 minutes, until the outside is crispy.

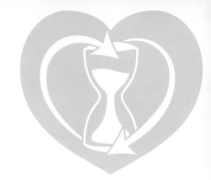

• Once the beetroots have cooked, set them aside to cool. Once cool, peel the skin off and place the beetroots in a blender.

• Drain the boiling potatoes and add them to the blender along with the lemon juice, cumin, garlic, coriander powder and coconut milk, plus some salt and pepper. Blend until smooth – if you find it's too thick at this point then add water until you reached your desired consistency.

• Place the soup into a saucepan and let it heat up to the perfect eating temperature.

• Pour the soup into bowls and sprinkle each bowl with the roast potato croutons!

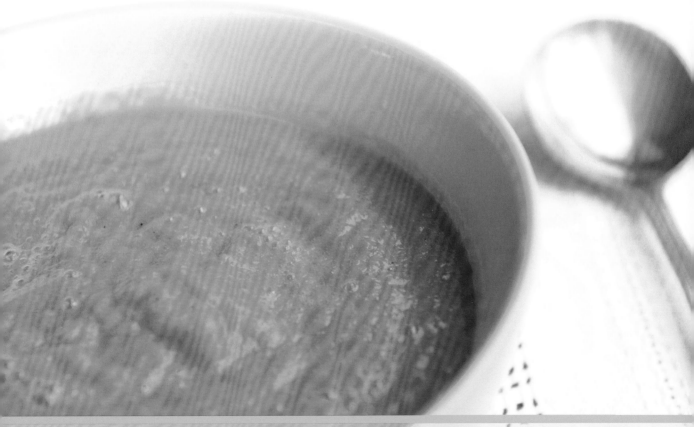

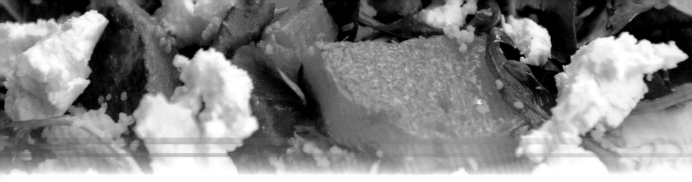

Butternut Squash & Couscous Salad

Ingredients

1 butternut squash, peeled and cubed
1 tbsp olive oil
1 bag wild rocket
4oz / 115g / $\frac{1}{2}$ cup couscous, cooked as per directions
2$\frac{1}{2}$oz / 75g / $\frac{1}{3}$ cup feta cheese, crumbled

FOR THE DRESSING:
1 tsp Dijon mustard
2 tbsps olive oil
Juice of $\frac{1}{2}$ lemon
Small bunch flat-leaved parsley
Small bunch mint
Salt and freshly ground black pepper

Preparation Method

• Steam the butternut squash for about 7 minutes.

• While it's cooking, make the dressing: finely chop the herbs and combine with the other ingredients.

• Prepare the couscous according to the directions.

• Heat the olive oil in a frying pan and fry the steamed butternut squash until golden.

• Fluff couscous with a fork and combine with the rocket and the roasted squash. Toss in the dressing, divide between two plates and crumble the feta cheese over the top.

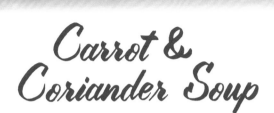

Carrot & Coriander Soup

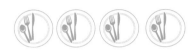 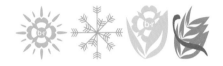

This is a delicious soup, quick and easy to make and very refreshing!

Ingredients

1 tbsp olive oil
3 large carrots, peeled and chopped
1 onion, chopped
1 pint / 570mls vegetable stock
Large bunch fresh coriander, chopped

Preparation Method

• Sauté the carrots and onion in the olive oil for a few minutes until the onion has softened a little.

• Add the vegetable stock and coriander to the pan. Bring to the boil, then simmer until the carrots are tender (10-12 minutes).

• Remove from heat and allow to cool slightly. Puree the soup until smooth.

Butternut Squash & Warm Tomato Salsa with Salad

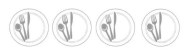 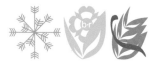

Ingredients

1 butternut squash (choose one with a long 'neck')
2 tbsps olive oil
1 red onion, finely sliced
1 clove garlic, minced
8oz / 225g / 1 cup mixed tomatoes, quartered (use red and yellow cherry, and baby plum)
16 black olives (approx.), stoned and sliced.
Small sprig basil leaves

FOR THE SALAD:
Rocket
Tomatoes
Spring onions
Radish
Pepper
Juice of a lemon
Salt and freshly ground black pepper

Preparation Method

• Preheat the oven to 190°C / 375°F / gas mark 5 and cover a baking tray with parchment paper.

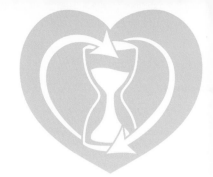

• Cut the squash in half, to separate the stem section from the round base. Peel the stem section and cut off eight rounds, about $^1/_4$ inch / $^1/_2$ cm thick.

• Arrange the rounds on the baking tray and brush with 1 tbsp of the oil, then bake for around 40 minutes, turning halfway through.

• When the squash is almost ready, make the salsa. Heat the oil in a pan and sauté the onion until softened. Add the garlic and cook for another 1-2 minutes.

• Add the tomatoes and olives and warm through for a couple of minutes.

• Spoon the warm salsa on top of the butternut squash rounds; garnish with the basil leaves.

• Serve with a fresh, crisp salad made from the ingredients listed, or those of your own choice, dressed with lemon juice and seasoned.

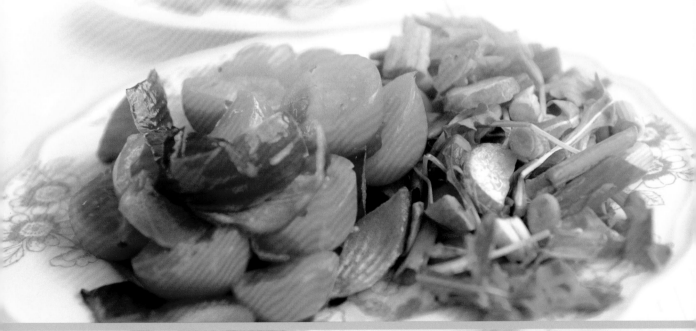

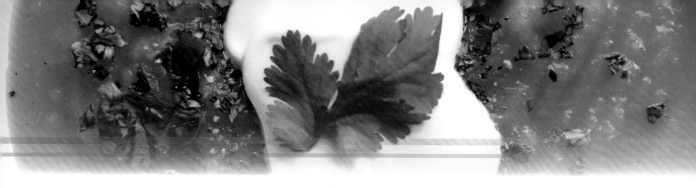

Carrot, Parsnip & Onion Soup

Ingredients

8oz / 225g / 1 cup carrot, peeled and diced
8oz / 225g / 1 cup parsnip, peeled and diced
1 onion, chopped
1 garlic clove, crushed
2 celery stalks, trimmed and chopped
1 bouquet garni
1 pint vegetable stock
Salt and pepper

TO SERVE:
Natural yogurt
Coriander leaves, chopped

Preparation Method

• Put all ingredients into a saucepan and bring to the boil. Reduce the heat and simmer for around 15 minutes, until the vegetables are tender.

• Remove from the heat and allow to cool slightly, then process the soup in a blender until smooth. (Discard the bouquet garni.)

• Return to the heat and season with salt and pepper.

• Serve with a swirl of natural yogurt and a sprinkling of chopped coriander.

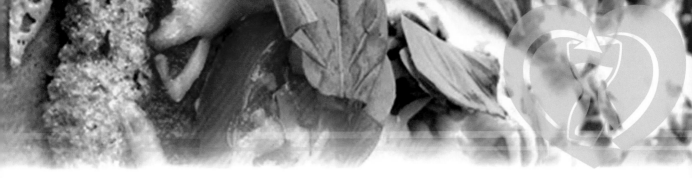

Cauliflower Pizza

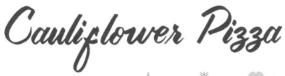

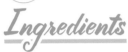

Ingredients

FOR THE PIZZA BASE:

1 cauliflower
8oz / 225g / 1 cup brown rice flour
2 tbsps chia seeds with 4fl oz / 120mls / $^1/_2$ cup water
$^1/_2$ mango
1 lemon
Dried herbs
Salt

TOPPING:
Add toppings of your choice, e.g. tomato puree, mushrooms, spinach, basil, tomatoes

Preparation Method

• Place the chia seeds in a cup with the water for 10-15 minutes, so that the mixture becomes gelatinous.

• Process the cauliflower in a blender, then place the mixture in a tea towel and squeeze out all the water, thoroughly.

• Combine all the pizza base ingredients together; flatten the dough out and place on a baking tray – oil the tray slightly to prevent sticking.

• Bake in the oven on 200°C / 390°F / gas mark 6 for about 25 minutes.

• Once cooked, add your topping and place back in the oven for a further 7 minutes.

A really delicious alternative to pizza – you will be so surprised how scrumptious it is!

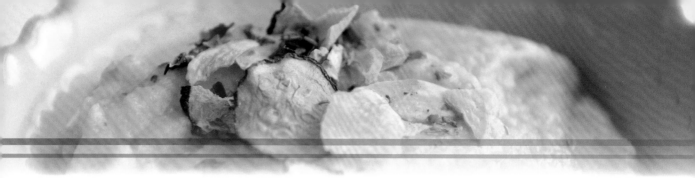

Cauliflower Soup

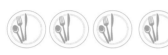

Ingredients

2 tbsps olive oil
2 shallots, chopped
4 spring onions, chopped
1 clove garlic, crushed
2 stalks celery, chopped
2 medium cauliflowers, broken into florets
1 tsp dried basil
$\frac{1}{2}$ tsp dried marjoram
$\frac{1}{2}$ tsp dried sage
Salt and freshly ground black pepper
$2\frac{1}{2}$ pints / 1.4 litres / 6 cups vegetable stock

Preparation Method

• Heat the oil in a large pan and cook the shallots and spring onions for 2 minutes.

• Add the garlic and celery and cook for another 2 minutes.

• Add the cauliflower and seasonings and cook for 3-4 minutes.

• Add the vegetable stock and bring to the boil. Simmer for around 15 minutes until the cauliflower is tender.

• Blend until smooth, then reheat and serve.

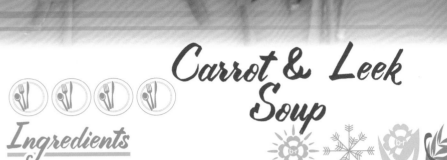

Carrot & Leek Soup

Ingredients

2lbs / 1kg / 4 cups carrots, sliced
2 large leeks, chopped
1 medium onion, chopped
2 stalks celery, chopped
2½ pints / 1.4 litres / 6 cups vegetable stock
3 tsps dried mixed herbs
GARNISH:
Chopped chives

Preparation Method

• In a large pan, bring the vegetable stock to the boil and add all ingredients. Simmer for 20 minutes or until vegetables are tender.

• Puree, reheat as necessary and serve garnished with chopped chives.

Chickpeas, Cherry Tomatoes & Rocket

Ingredients

1 bag rocket
1 tin (15oz / 400g) chickpeas, drained and rinsed
12 cherry tomatoes, quartered
Juice of ½ lemon
Salt and freshly ground black pepper

Preparation Method

• Mix the rocket, chickpeas and tomatoes, dress with the lemon juice and season with salt and pepper.

Celeriac Salad

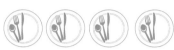 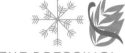

YOU WILL NEED A VEGETABLE JUICER FOR THE DRESSING!

Ingredients

1 celeriac, peeled
2 anchovies, chopped
2 apples, chopped
A handful of chopped parsley
10$\frac{1}{2}$oz / 300g / 1$\frac{1}{4}$ cups smoked salmon
FOR THE DRESSING:
2oz / 55g / $\frac{1}{4}$ cup celeriac juice
1oz / 28g / 0.12 cup lemon juice
1 garlic clove
1 tsp salt
1 tsp black pepper
1 tsp cinnamon
1 tsp turmeric
1 tbsp olive oil
1 tsp apple cider vinegar

Preparation Method

• Use a vegetable peeler to slice the celeriac into long ribbons. Stop at the soft centre and throw this away.

• In a large bowl, mix together the ribbons of celeriac, anchovies, apples and parsley.

• Put all the ingredients for the dressing into a vegetable juicer and process.

• Divide the salad between four plates and drizzle the dressing on the top.

• Serve with the smoked salmon.

Celeriac is rich in vitamins A, C, K and E, and is great for the digestion!

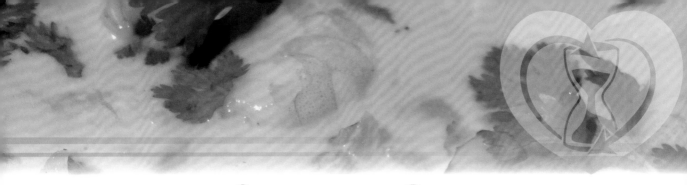

Coconut & Prawn Soup

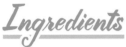

Ingredients

1 tbsp coconut oil
1 onion, finely chopped
1 clove garlic, minced or crushed
½ tbsp grated fresh root ginger
¼ red chilli, minced
1 tsp finely chopped lemongrass
2/3 pint / 350mls water
6fl oz / 165mls coconut milk
1 tbsp fish sauce
8oz / 225g / 1 cup uncooked prawns
1 small pak choi, finely shredded
Juice of ½ lime
Salt and freshly ground black pepper
Fresh coriander, chopped

Preparation Method

• Heat the oil in a large saucepan over a medium heat then add the onion, garlic, ginger, chilli, and lemongrass and sauté for 3-4 minutes.

• Add in the water, coconut milk and fish sauce, and bring to the boil.

• Reduce the heat and add the prawns and the pak choi; simmer gently for 2-3 minutes, until the prawns are pink and cooked through.

• Stir in the lime juice, and season to taste with salt and freshly ground black pepper.

• Serve garnished with chopped fresh coriander.

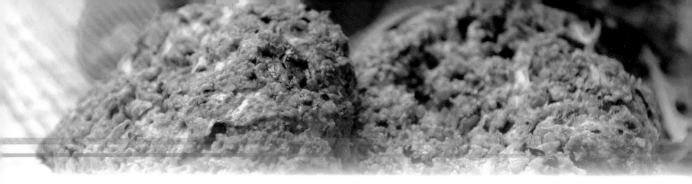

Courgette Burgers

Ingredients

1lb / 500g / 2 cups peas
1 small courgette
8oz / 225g / 1 cup ground flaxseeds
8oz / 225g / 1 cup quinoa
1 lime
1 tbsp of apple cider vinegar
1 tbsp of tahini
Handful of fresh coriander
Salt to taste
GARNISH:
Hummus
Slices of avocado
Slices of tomato
Rocket / butter lettuce

Preparation Method

• Cook the quinoa according to the directions.

• Meanwhile cook the peas in a pan of water.

• When the peas are cooked, process them in a blender to form a paste. Transfer to a mixing bowl

• Grate the courgette and add to the bowl along with the juiced lime, apple cider vinegar, tahini, finely chopped coriander, ground flaxseeds and salt.

• Add the cooked quinoa to the bowl and mix everything well. Mould the mixture into patties, place on a baking tray and bake for 20 minutes at 180°C / 350°F / gas mark 4.

• Serve with salad and hummus.

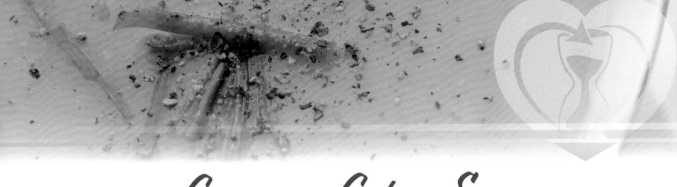

Cream of Celery Soup

MAKES THREE GENEROUS SERVINGS; LEFTOVERS MAY BE FROZEN.

Ingredients

1 tbsp olive oil
6oz / 170g / ¾ cup onion, finely chopped
2 cloves garlic, crushed or finely chopped
1 heaped tbsp vegetable bouillon powder dissolved in 1½ pints / 850mls of boiling water
12oz / 340g / 1½ cups potato, chopped
1 large head celery, chopped (reserve one stalk)
1 tbsp cornflour, dissolved in 1 tbsp cold water
¼ pint / 140mls soya milk
Salt and freshly ground black pepper

Preparation Method

• Heat the oil in a heavy based pan and sauté the onion until soft (about 2 minutes). Add the garlic and sauté for a further minute

• Add the bouillon, the potatoes and the celery, bring to the boil, then simmer for around 20 minutes until vegetables are tender.

• Allow to cool slightly, then puree in a blender until smooth.

• Return the soup to the pan and bring to a simmer. Add the cornflour and water and stir constantly until thickened.

• Slice the reserved celery stalk very finely and add to the soup. Stir in the soya milk and season with salt and freshly ground black pepper. Heat thoroughly before serving.

Filled Potato Shells & Salad

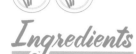

Ingredients

2 large baking potatoes
2 tsps olive oil
1 onion, chopped
4oz / 115g / ½ cup cheese, grated or chopped into small pieces (cheddar works well, as does adding a little mozzarella to the mix)
Sun-dried tomato, chopped (optional)
Jalapenos, chopped (optional)
Salt and freshly ground black pepper

FOR THE SALAD:
Little gem lettuce
Cherry tomatoes
Cucumber
Peppers
Lemon juice

If you wish you can reserve a little cheese to sprinkle on the top!

Preparation Method

• Bake the potatoes and cut in half. Scoop out the middle, leaving around ¼ inch next to the skin.

• Fry the onion in 1 tsp olive oil until soft; set aside.

• Season the potato with salt and pepper, add 1 tsp olive oil and mash until smooth. Stir in the cheese and fried onions, plus the sun-dried tomatoes and jalapenos, if using, and mix thoroughly.

• Spoon the mixture back into the shells and put back into the hot oven for around 10 minutes until the cheese has melted and the potatoes are hot.

• Chop up the salad vegetables, mix in a bowl and dress with the lemon juice. Serve with the filled potato shells.

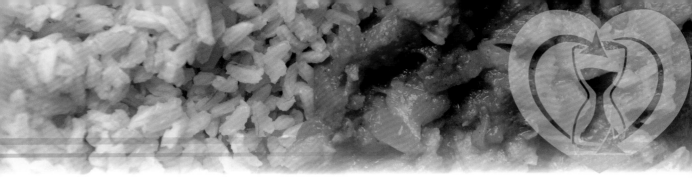

Fish Curry

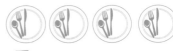

Ingredients

12oz / 340g / 1¹/₂ cups basmati rice
1 tbsp coconut oil
1 large onion, chopped
1 garlic clove, crushed
2 tsps curry powder (or however much you prefer)
1 tsp garam masala
1 tsp ground cumin
1 tin (15oz / 400g) tomatoes
¹/₂ pint / 285mls vegetable stock
4 x white fish fillets, skinned and cut into chunks

Preparation Method

• The curry will only take 10-12 minutes to cook, so first put the rice on. Time things so that the rice and curry are ready together.

• Heat the oil in a large, heavy based pan and sauté the onion for 2-3 minutes; add the garlic and cook for another couple of minutes. Add the spices and fry for 1-2 minutes longer.

• Add the tomatoes and stock to the pan and bring to the boil. Reduce the heat until the sauce is simmering gently.

• Add the fish to the curry sauce and cook for 4-5 minutes. It's ready when the fish flakes easily. Serve the fish curry immediately, over the rice.

Fish Stew

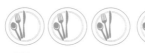

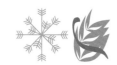

Ingredients

Vegetable stock
1lb / 450g / 2 cups white fish
1 tbsp olive oil
1 chopped onion
2 tins (15oz / 400g) chopped tomatoes
1 handful of fresh parsley
Salt and pepper to taste

Preparation Method

• Place the fish in stock in an ovenproof dish and bake in the oven for 10-15 minutes on 200°C / 390°F / gas mark 6.

• Heat the oil in a deep frying pan and fry the onion until soft.

• Add the tomatoes and fresh parsley.

• Add the fish and stock to the frying pan and season with salt and pepper

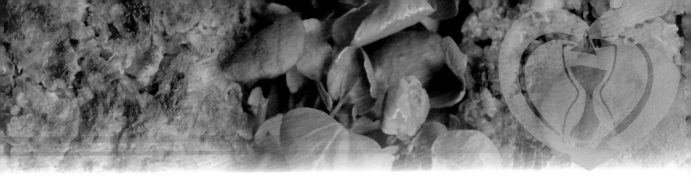

Fishcakes with Sweet Potato

MAKES 8 PATTIES

Ingredients

1 large sweet potato
8oz / 225g / 1 cup quinoa
1 large tin (418g) wild red salmon
1 tsp chilli flakes
1 handful fresh parsley, chopped
1 handful coriander, chopped
1 handful chives, chopped
3 spring onions, chopped
Zest of 1 lemon
1 egg
2 tbsp coconut oil

Preparation Method

- Preheat the oven to 180°C / 350°F / gas mark 4 and bake sweet potato for 45 minutes.
- Cook quinoa in boiling water for 10 minutes.
- Combine salmon, chilli, parsley, coriander, pepper, chives, lemon and spring onions in a bowl, mix in the cooked quinoa.
- Once the sweet potato is cooked, remove skin and add to the mixture.
- Crack an egg into the mixture and combine thoroughly.
- Shape mixture into 8 palm-sized patties.
- Add oil to a pan and cook for 3-5 minutes each side.
- Serve with salad.

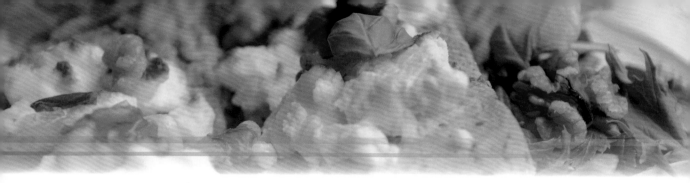

Goat's Cheese on Toast & Walnut Salad

USE SLICES OF NUT BREAD

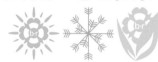

Ingredients

7 oz / 200g / scant 1 cup goat's cheese
5^{1}/$_{2}$oz / 150g / ^{2}/$_{3}$ cup rocket, spinach and lettuce
5^{1}/$_{2}$oz / 150g / ^{2}/$_{3}$ cup walnuts
1 handful flat-leaved parsley
1 handful basil
1 clove garlic, crushed
3 tbsp apple cider vinegar
4 tbsp walnut oil

Preparation Method

• Toast one side of your bread, place goat's cheese on the other side and grill until melted.

• Blend the oil, vinegar and garlic for the dressing.

• Combine the greens, basil and parsley on your plate with the cheese on toast and drizzle over the dressing.

Goat's cheese has far fewer calories than cow's cheese. Goat's cheese contains more vitamin D and vitamin K, thiamine, and niacin. It's also a good source of riboflavin (a B vitamin) and phosphorus!

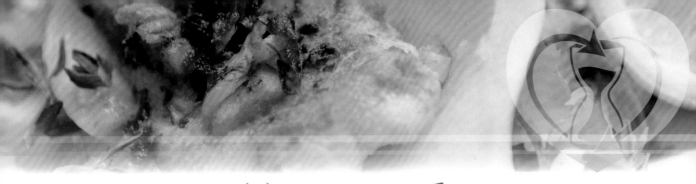

Halibut & Fennel Salad

Ingredients

1 tsp ground coriander
$\frac{1}{2}$ tsp ground cumin
1 tbsp extra virgin olive oil
2 garlic cloves
4 x 6oz / 170g halibut fillets
1 tsp coconut oil

SALAD INGREDIENTS:
1 small fennel bulb, chopped
$\frac{1}{2}$ red onion, chopped
2 tbsp fresh lemon juice
1 bunch chopped flat-leaved parsley
1 handful thyme leaves

Preparation Method

• Combine coriander, cumin and oil with garlic cloves, and rub on fish.

• Heat 1 tsp coconut oil in a pan and add fish.

• Cook for around 5 minutes on each side.

• Combine salad ingredients and serve with fish.

The anethole in fennel has repeatedly been shown to reduce inflammation and also helps prevent the occurrence of cancer.

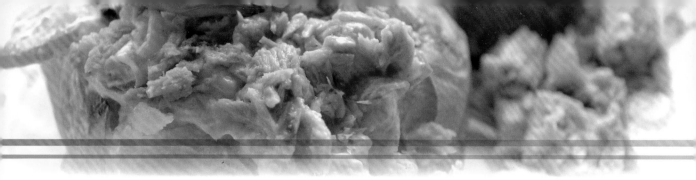

Jacket Potato & Salad

 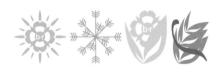

Ingredients

1 can tuna
1 red pepper
8 spring onions
1 sweetcorn cob (cooked and sliced)
1 tbsp crème fraîche
1 jacket potato
½ tbsp coconut oil

Preparation Method

• Mix together all ingredients apart from the jacket potato and coconut oil to make a delicious salad.

• Place the oil in the potato to fluff up and serve with the salad.

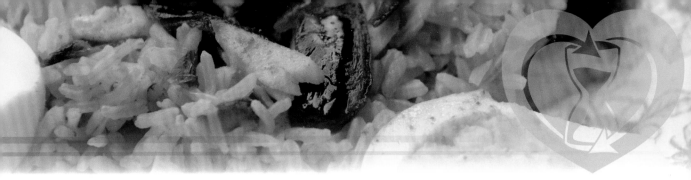

Kedgeree

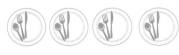

Ingredients

4oz / 115g / $\frac{1}{2}$ cup brown rice
8oz / 225g / 1 cup smoked haddock fillets
4 eggs
1 tsp coconut oil
$\frac{1}{2}$ onion, finely chopped
1 tsp curry powder
Small handful fresh parsley, chopped
$\frac{1}{2}$ lemon, juiced

Preparation Method

• Put the rice on to cook.

• After about 10 minutes, put the eggs on to hard boil.

• Next put the haddock in a large frying pan with just enough water to cover. Bring to simmering point, then simmer for 2-3 minutes, until tender. Drain, skin and flake the haddock, discarding any bones.

• Melt the coconut oil in a saucepan and fry the onion over a low heat until tender, then add the curry powder and cook for 1-2 minutes. Add the cooked rice and fish. Season well. Stir over a moderate heat for about 5 minutes until hot, then stir in the parsley and lemon juice.

• Meanwhile, shell the eggs, quarter and arrange on top of the kedgeree to serve.

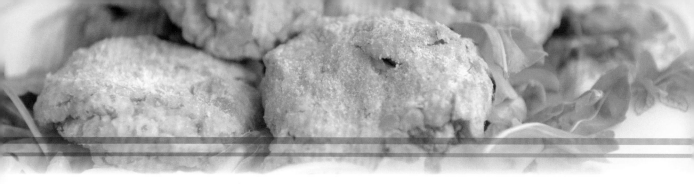

Lentil Burgers with Salad

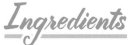

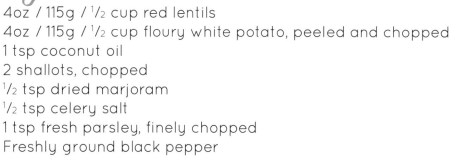

Ingredients

4oz / 115g / $\frac{1}{2}$ cup red lentils
4oz / 115g / $\frac{1}{2}$ cup floury white potato, peeled and chopped
1 tsp coconut oil
2 shallots, chopped
$\frac{1}{2}$ tsp dried marjoram
$\frac{1}{2}$ tsp celery salt
1 tsp fresh parsley, finely chopped
Freshly ground black pepper
3-4 tbsps rice flour

Preparation Method

• Cook the lentils in water, drain and set aside.

• Boil or steam the potatoes until cooked, then mash and set aside.

• Sauté the shallots in the oil until soft.

• Preheat the oven to 180°C / 350°F / gas mark 4 and line a baking sheet with baking parchment.

• Combine all ingredients thoroughly, then divide into four equal portions. Shape into patties and coat in the rice flour, then put on the baking sheet.

• Bake in the oven for 20-25 minutes, turning halfway through the cooking time.

• Serve with a nice crispy salad

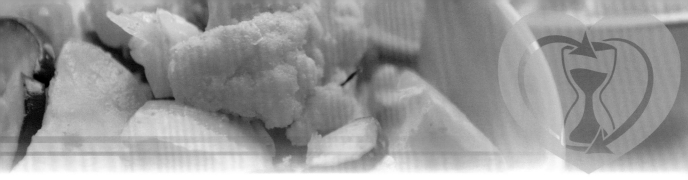

Mixed Vegetable Curry

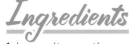

Ingredients

1 tsp olive oil
1 large onion, chopped
4 cloves garlic, crushed
$1/2$ tsp turmeric
$1/2$ tsp ground cumin
$1/2$ tsp ground ginger
1 tsp medium curry powder
1lb 10oz / 750g / $3^{1}/_{4}$ cups sweet potato, chopped
1 medium cauliflower, broken into florets
4oz / 115g / $1/2$ cup green beans, halved
2 carrots. sliced
2 courgettes, sliced
6fl oz / 170mls vegetable stock or water
Salt and freshly ground black pepper
10oz / 280g / $1^{1}/_{4}$ cups basmati rice

Preparation Method

• Sauté the onions and garlic in the olive oil for 3-4 minutes.

• Add the spices and cook gently for another minute.

• Stir in the prepared vegetables and stir, making sure they are all coated with the spices.

• Add the liquid, season with salt and pepper, and cook, uncovered, for 15-20 minutes until the vegetables are tender.

• While the curry cooks, cook the basmati rice. Serve the curry on a bed of rice.

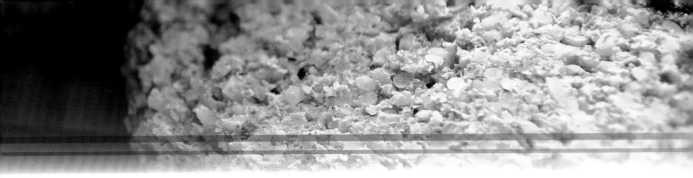

Nut Bread

Ingredients

9oz / 250g of almonds
9oz / 250g quinoa flakes or brown rice
10½oz / 300g pumpkin seeds
7oz / 200g sunflower seeds
2 tbsp chia seeds
3 heaped tbsp psyllium husk powder
2 tbsp dried mixed herbs

Preparation Method

• Place the almonds, quinoa flakes and half the pumpkin seeds in a food processor and process until smooth.

• Place the mix in a bowl with the remaining pumpkin seeds and the sunflower seeds, chia seeds, psyllium husk, dried herbs and salt to taste.

• Add 2½ glasses of cold water. Let the mixture sit for an hour.

• Heat the oven to 180°C / 350°F / gas mark 4.

• Once the mixture is really firm, grease the base of a loaf tin with coconut or olive oil, pour the mixture in and press it down with a spoon. Bake in the oven for 40 minutes to an hour, until the top begins to brown and you can pull a knife out of the middle without any of the mixture sticking to it. Finally, slice, smother on your favourite toppings and enjoy.

Storing the bread in the fridge makes it last longer, and you can freeze it, too.

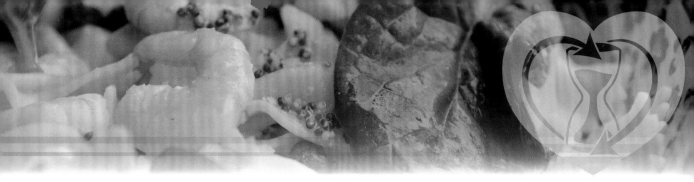

Pasta Prawn Salad

MAKE THIS RECIPE GLUTEN-FREE BY USING GLUTEN-FREE PASTA.

Ingredients

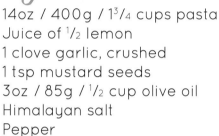

14oz / 400g / 1³/₄ cups pasta
Juice of ¹/₂ lemon
1 clove garlic, crushed
1 tsp mustard seeds
3oz / 85g / ¹/₂ cup olive oil
Himalayan salt
Pepper
12oz / 340g / 1¹/₂ cups cooked peeled prawns
7oz / 200g / scant 1 cup chopped fresh spinach
3oz / 85g / ¹/₃ cup tinned cannellini beans, drained and rinsed
1 red onion, finely chopped
2 tbsps chopped capers

Preparation Method

• Cook pasta according to directions.

• Combine juice, mustard seeds, oil and garlic in a small bowl and whisk. Stir in salt and pepper.

• Combine the rest of the ingredients in a bowl and pour the dressing on the top to serve.

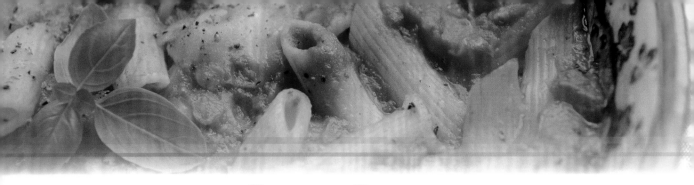

Penne Pasta Bake

MAKE THIS RECIPE GLUTEN-FREE BY USING GLUTEN-FREE PASTA.

Ingredients

1 tin (15oz / 400g) chopped tomatoes
$^3/_4$ pint / 425mls vegetable stock or water
1 tsp dried oregano
1 tsp dried basil
Tomato puree
1 small tin anchovies, chopped
Around 1 dozen black olives, sliced
1 heaped tbsp capers (optional)
8oz / 225g / 2 cups penne pasta
$2^1/_2$oz / 75g / $^1/_3$ cup grated mozzarella cheese

Preparation Method

• Preheat the oven to 210°C / 410°F / gas mark 6.

• Add the tomatoes and stock or water to an ovenproof dish (with a lid). Add the dried herbs and a generous dollop of tomato puree, and stir until thoroughly mixed. (If you wish, you could use your wine allowance in the dish, in which case add it at this stage and reduce the amount of stock or water accordingly.)

• Add the anchovies, olives, capers (if using), and pasta. Sprinkle the mozzarella on the top. Fit the lid and bake in the oven for 20-30 minutes, until the pasta is cooked.

Note that the cheese will help to thicken the sauce.

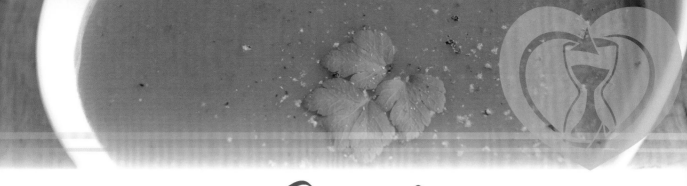

Pepper & Paprika Soup

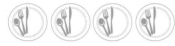

Ingredients

2 tbsps coconut oil
1 small onion, diced
2 large red peppers, deseeded and diced
1-2 fresh green chillies
2 tsps paprika
$\frac{1}{2}$ tsp ground cardamom
1 tsp Himalayan salt
4oz / 115g / $\frac{1}{2}$ cup pistachios
17fl ozs / 475mls / 2 cups vegetable stock
2 tbsps fromage frais
2oz / 55g / $\frac{1}{4}$ cup finely torn basil

Preparation Method

• Heat the oil in a large saucepan. Add onion, peppers and chilli and cook for 3-5 minutes. Add paprika, salt and cardamom and cook, stirring, until the spices are very fragrant – 1 to 2 minutes.

• Add pistachios and vegetable stock. Stir and bring to a boil. Reduce the heat and simmer for 20 to 25 minutes.

• Transfer the soup to a blender and blend.

• When ready to serve, whisk in fromage frais and sprinkle basil on top.

One teaspoon of paprika has 37% of the recommended daily intake of vitamin A; it also contains vitamin B6, iron and capsaicin.

Pumpkin Soup

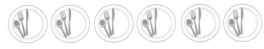

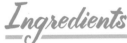

Ingredients

2¼lbs / 1kg / 4 ⅓ cups Jap pumpkin
1lb / 500g / 2 cups carrots
2 tbsp olive oil
Good pinch of sea salt and black pepper to taste
½ tsp ground cinnamon
1¾ pints / 1L water or vegetable stock
1 tsp fresh grated ginger (optional)

Preparation Method

• Preheat your oven to 200°C / 390°F / gas mark 6.

• Peel and chop pumpkin into small chunks and place on a lined baking tray.

• Wash carrots and chop roughly, leaving the skin on. Place on a separate lined baking tray.

• Drizzle the olive oil between the 2 trays. Season each tray with sea salt, pepper and a little cinnamon. Mix the oil and seasoning through the vegetables with your fingers.

• Roast for 40-45 minutes or until vegetables are cooked through and caramelised.

• Combine pumpkin and carrot in a high performance blender like a Vitamix. Add about ¾ of the water, and ginger, if using. Blend until smooth.

• Add more water to adjust consistency.

• Serve soup hot and feel the nourishment.

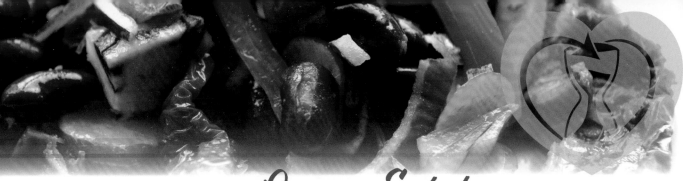

Quinoa Salad

Ingredients

9oz / 250g / 1 cup cooked quinoa
2 celery sticks
2 spring onions
1lb / 500g / 2 cups grapes
1 lime, juiced
2 tbsp oil
1 handful mint
1 handful basil
Pinch of salt

Preparation Method

• Place all ingredients in a bowl and mix together for a very tasty and filling salad.

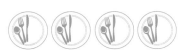

Red Salad

Ingredients

Red salad leaves, e.g. lollo rosso
1 red onion, thinly sliced
1 red pepper, cut into strips
6 radishes, sliced
2oz / 60g / $\frac{1}{2}$ cup sun-dried tomatoes (not in oil), sliced
1 tin (15oz / 400g) red kidney beans, drained and rinsed
Juice of a lime
Salt and freshly ground black pepper

Preparation Method

• Combine all the salad vegetables with the sun-dried tomatoes and the kidney beans.

• Dress with the lime juice and season with salt and pepper.

Chapter 6: Recipes
Lunch & Supper

Quinoa Falafels & Tahini Sauce

Ingredients

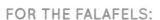

FOR THE FALAFELS:
4oz / 115g / ½ cup quinoa
8oz / 225g / 1 cup chopped carrot
4oz / 115g / ½ cup sliced green onions (about 3)
3 tbsp chopped parsley
1 tin (15oz / 400g) chickpeas (garbanzo beans)
2 eggs
2 tbsp fresh lemon juice
1 tsp cumin
2 tsp coriander
2 tbsp toasted sesame seeds
2 cloves garlic
Salt and freshly ground black pepper
2 tbsp olive oil
FOR THE TAHINI SAUCE:
8oz / 225g / 1 cup plain yogurt
2oz / 55 g / ¼ cup tahini
1 tbsp lemon zest
Fresh chives to taste
Salt and freshly ground black pepper
TO SERVE:
1 English cucumber, cut into matchsticks

Preparation Method

• In a small saucepan, bring 8fl oz / 227mls / 1 cup water to a boil. Add quinoa, cover, and reduce heat to low. Cook until liquid is absorbed, about 12 minutes. Set aside to cool for now.

• In a bowl, whisk together the yogurt, tahini, lemon zest, a pinch of salt and

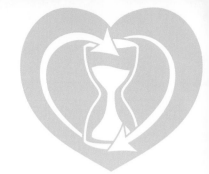

pepper, and chives if you have them. Cover and put in the fridge.

• In a blender or food processor, pulse the carrots and parsley. Add the green onion, chickpeas, sesame seeds, lemon juice, eggs, garlic, coriander and cumin. Season with salt and freshly ground pepper. Pulse until roughly combined, add quinoa, and give it another few pulses. (I prefer it chunky.) Taste for seasonings. Allow to set in fridge for an hour. It will be fine resting overnight if you really like to plan ahead.

• Heat a nonstick pan* over a medium high heat with 1 tbsp of the oil. Scoop the mixture out in roughly 2 tbsp size portions, roll and flatten into patties. Sear them in the saucepan for about 3 minutes on each side, with a slight press of the spatula between to thin the patty a bit. Use the remaining oil when the pan becomes dry, about the third batch.

I ate mine at room temperature over some matchstick cucumbers, with a drizzle of the yogurt tahini sauce on top. You could put them in mini pitas and they could be a neat veg appetizer. I love mini things!

*Using a nonstick pan will allow you to use less oil to keep the falafels from sticking. You need some oil to create a crust, but you are not 'frying' them.

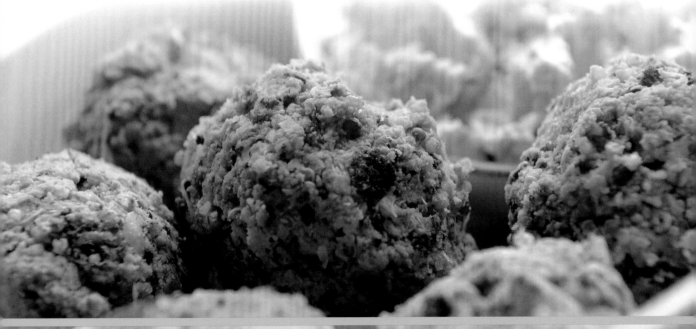

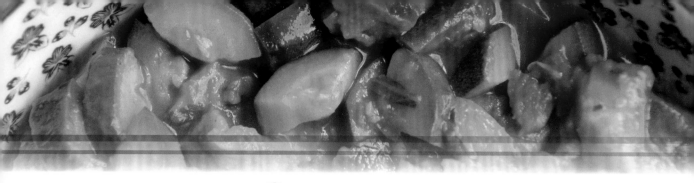

Ratatouille

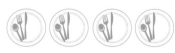

Ingredients

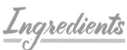

1 tbsp olive oil
1 large onion, chopped
2 cloves garlic, crushed
1 courgette, chopped
1 red pepper, chopped
1 aubergine, roughly chopped
1 x 15oz / 400g can chopped tomatoes
3 tbsp fresh basil, chopped
Salt and freshly ground black pepper

Preparation Method

• Sauté the onions and garlic in the olive oil for 3-4 minutes.

• Stir in the courgettes, peppers and aubergine, and cook for a further 5 minutes until golden.

• Add the tomatoes and half the basil, cover and cook over a low heat until the vegetables are tender (about half an hour). Season, and sprinkle with the remaining chopped basil to serve.

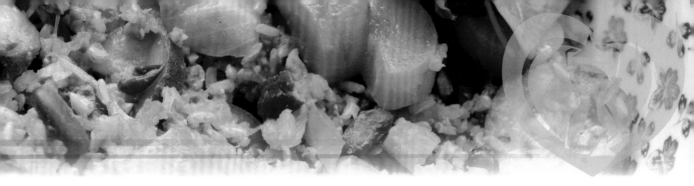

Rice & Veg with Beans

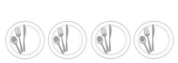

Ingredients

1 tbsp olive oil
2 onions, chopped
2 garlic cloves, thinly sliced
12oz / 340g / 1½ cups brown rice
1tbsp turmeric
1 pint vegetable stock or water
½ pint / 285mls tomato juice
2 large carrots, peeled and diced
1 parsnip, peeled and diced
2 courgettes, sliced
1 red pepper, deseeded and chopped
1 tin (15oz / 400g) cannellini beans
Salt and freshly ground black pepper

TO SERVE:
1 handful fresh flat-leaved parsley, finely chopped
Parmesan, finely grated (optional)

Preparation Method

• Heat the oil in a large saucepan over a medium heat. Add the onion and garlic and sauté for 4-5 minutes.

• Add the turmeric and cook for a minute, then add the rice and coat thoroughly with the oil and turmeric.

• Add the tomato juice and stock or water, bring to the boil, reduce the heat, cover, and simmer for 15 minutes.

• Add the carrot, parsnip, courgette, pepper and beans, and cook for a further 10 minutes, until the vegetables are tender.

• Remove from the heat and allow to stand, covered, for 5 minutes. Fluff the rice up with a fork, season with salt and pepper, and serve.

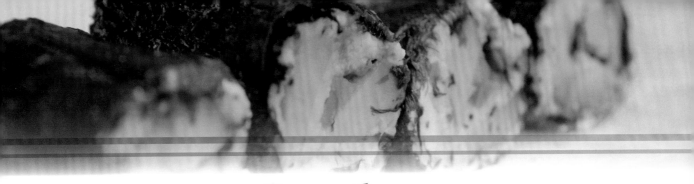

Rice Free Vegetable Sushi

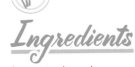

Ingredients

1 nori sheet
1 egg
1 tbsp mung bean sprouts
2 tbsp feta cheese
$\frac{1}{2}$ avocado

Preparation Method

• Lay nori sheet on a sushi bamboo mat.

• Cut the sheet in half.

• Dampen the sheets with some water.

• Make the omelette: whisk the egg, then add the mung beans and feta cheese. Cook in an omelette pan for 4-5 minutes.

• Place the omelette and avocado on the nori sheet, and roll up.

• Cut the roll into 2 inch sections and serve.

Nori seaweed is incredibly rich in nutrients – it is especially high in iron and omega 3; it also helps lower cholesterol.

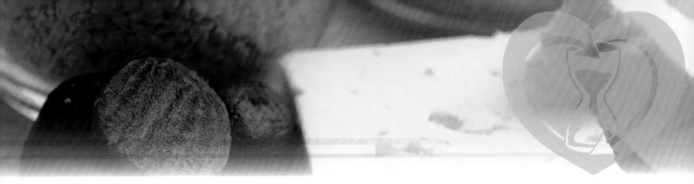

Rice, Lentil & Beetroot Salad with Goat's Cheese

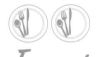 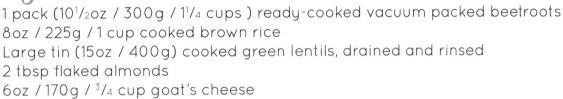

Ingredients

1 pack (10$\frac{1}{2}$oz / 300g / 1$\frac{1}{4}$ cups) ready-cooked vacuum packed beetroots
8oz / 225g / 1 cup cooked brown rice
Large tin (15oz / 400g) cooked green lentils, drained and rinsed
2 tbsp flaked almonds
6oz / 170g / $\frac{3}{4}$ cup goat's cheese

FOR THE DRESSING:
2 tbsp apple cider vinegar
1 tsp Dijon mustard
1 tbsp extra virgin olive oil
Drizzle of honey
$\frac{1}{4}$ tsp dried mint
Salt and freshly ground black pepper

Preparation Method

• Cut the beetroots into wedges.

• Whisk together the vinegar, mustard, olive oil, honey, chopped mint and seasoning to make the dressing.

• Combine the rice and lentils in a bowl.

• Add the beetroots, then pour over the dressing and toss to combine. Transfer to a plates or bowls and sprinkle over the flaked almonds and feta cheese to serve.

Roasted Red Pepper Soup

Ingredients

4 red peppers
Olive oil
2 pints / 1135mls vegetable stock or water
2 cloves garlic, crushed
1 large red onion, roughly chopped
1 large carrot, roughly chopped
2 sticks celery, roughly chopped
1 tin (15oz / 400g) chopped tomatoes
Large handful of fresh basil leaves
Salt and freshly ground black pepper

Preparation Method

● Preheat the oven to 200°C / 390°F / gas mark 6 and line a baking sheet with baking paper.

● Remove the stalks from the peppers, cut into quarters and remove the seeds. Brush with olive oil and put on the baking tray. Bake for 5 minutes or so until the skins begin to char. Remove from the oven and when they are cool enough to handle put them into a plastic bag and allow to cool.

● Meanwhile put the stock and the prepared vegetables into a saucepan and bring to the boil; cook for 5-6 minutes. Turn down the heat and simmer for 10 minutes.

● By now the peppers should be cool. Take them from the bag and peel off the charred skin. It should come away easily. Roughly chop the flesh.

● Add the chopped peppers and the tinned tomatoes to the saucepan. Simmer for a further 5 minutes or so until the vegetables are tender. Remove from the heat and add the fresh basil. Allow to cool slightly, then puree until smooth. Reheat as necessary and season with salt and pepper.

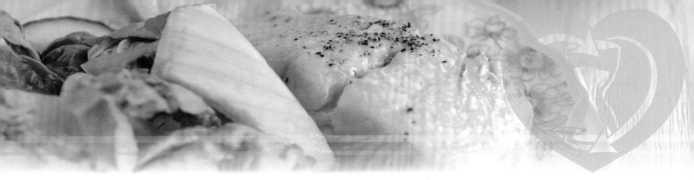

Salmon Steaks & Green Salad

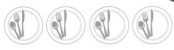

Ingredients

4 salmon steaks
Juice of a lemon
Salt and freshly ground black pepper
2 heads little gem lettuce, washed, dried and chopped.
1/2 cucumber, finely sliced
2 stalks celery, finely sliced
1 bulb fennel, finely sliced
Lemon juice

Preparation Method

• Place the salmon steaks in a baking dish lined with parchment paper, sprinkle with lemon juice and season with salt and pepper.

• Bake, uncovered, at 200°C / 390°F / gas mark 6 for 15-20 minutes or until the fish flakes easily with a fork.

• Meanwhile, prepare the salad: combine all ingredients and dress with lemon juice.

• Serve the salmon steaks with the green salad.

Smoked Tofu Stir Fry

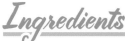

Ingredients

8oz / 225g / 1 cup brown rice
2 tbsp coconut oil
8oz / 225g / 1 cup smoked tofu, cubed
2 cloves garlic, crushed
2 tsp ginger, finely chopped
6oz / 170g / $^3/_4$ cup carrots, julienned
1 green pepper, cut into thin strips
1 red pepper, cut into thin strips
3$^1/_2$oz / 100g / 0.4 cup baby corn, cut in half lengthwise
4$^1/_2$oz / 130g / $^1/_2$ cup chestnut mushrooms, sliced thinly
3$^1/_2$oz / 100g / 0.4 cup green beans, cut on the diagonal

FOR THE SAUCE:
2 tbsps light soy sauce
1 tbsp apple juice
1 tbsp sweet chilli sauce (no added sugar, e.g. Trinity Hill Farms)
1 tbsp toasted sesame oil
1 tsp tomato puree

Preparation Method

• Put the rice on to cook; if it's ready early, keep it warm until your stir fry is cooked.

• Combine all the ingredients for the sauce and mix well.

• Prepare the tofu and the vegetables in advance.

• Heat the coconut oil in a wok. Add the tofu, ginger and garlic and stir-fry for 1-2 minutes.

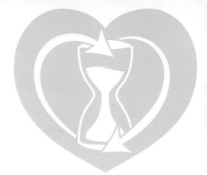

- Add the carrots and pepper to the wok, and fry for another 2-3 minutes.

- Add the mushrooms and baby corn, and cook for a few more minutes.

- Finally, add the green beans, and stir-fry for 1 minute until they turn bright green.

- Pour the sauce over the vegetables in the wok, stir through and cook for a couple more minutes.

- Serve immediately, with the rice.

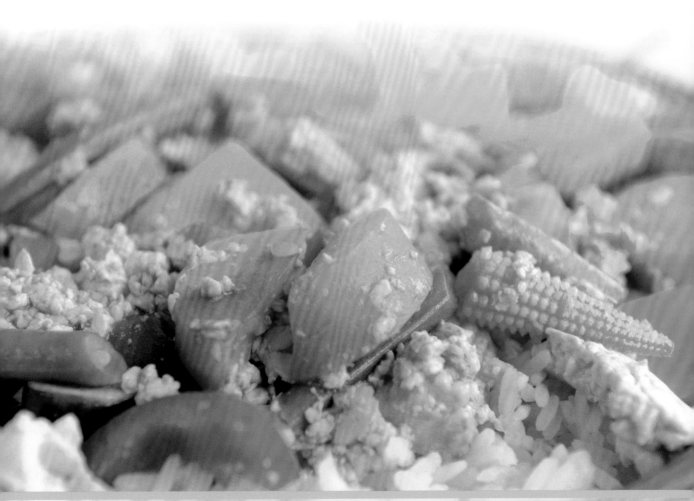

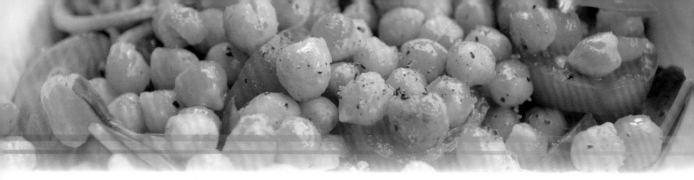

Spicy Baked Chickpea Salad

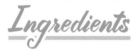

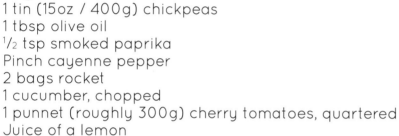

Ingredients

1 tin (15oz / 400g) chickpeas
1 tbsp olive oil
$\frac{1}{2}$ tsp smoked paprika
Pinch cayenne pepper
2 bags rocket
1 cucumber, chopped
1 punnet (roughly 300g) cherry tomatoes, quartered
Juice of a lemon
Salt and freshly ground black pepper

Preparation Method

• Pre-heat the oven to 200°C / 390°F / gas mark 6, and line a baking sheet with baking parchment.

• Combine the olive oil and spices in a bowl. Wash and dry the chickpeas, then add them to the bowl and make sure they're evenly coated. Spread out in a single layer on the baking sheet. Bake for around 30 minutes, until golden and crispy – shake the tray after about 15 minutes.

• Just before they finish cooking, chop the cucumber and tomatoes into small pieces and mix in a bowl with the rocket. Dress with the lemon juice and season with salt and pepper. Divide between four bowls.

• Share the chickpeas evenly, sprinkling them over the salad, then serve.

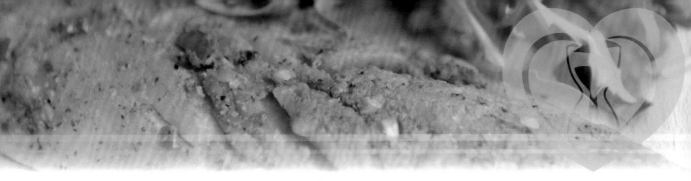

Spicy Mackerel with Green Salad

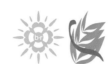

Ingredients

1 tin mackerel in curry sauce
Rocket
Spring onions
Cucumber
Celery
Lemon juice
Salt and pepper

Preparation Method

• Chop the vegetables and mix with the rocket to make the green salad. Dress with lemon juice and season with salt and pepper.

• Serve with the mackerel, mashed if you like.

If you prefer, use mackerel in tomato sauce.

Spicy Bean Burgers with Salad

Ingredients

1 tsp olive oil
1 onion, finely chopped
1 small carrot, grated
$\frac{1}{2}$ green pepper, finely chopped
1 clove garlic, crushed or finely chopped
$\frac{1}{2}$ tsp dried oregano
$\frac{1}{2}$ tsp (or to your taste) chilli powder
1 tin (15oz / 400g) red kidney beans
Salt and black pepper
Rice flour

FOR THE SALAD:
Rocket
Tomatoes
Spring onions
Radish
Pepper

Preparation Method

• Add the olive oil to a non-stick pan and sauté the onion, carrot and chilli for about 5 minutes.

• Add the garlic, oregano and chilli powder and cook for another minute, then remove from the heat.

• Drain the beans and roughly mash them, adding salt and pepper to season, then mix thoroughly with the cooked vegetables.

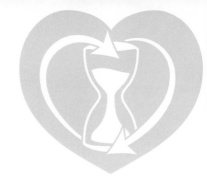

- Preheat the oven to 200°C / 390°F / gas mark 6.

- Sprinkle flour onto a flat surface, and lightly flour your hands. Divide the mixture into 4 equal parts on the floured surface and shape them into patties, making sure they're fully coated in flour.

- Lightly oil a baking tray and place the patties on it. Bake them in the oven for 20 minutes, turning halfway through the cooking time.

- Serve with a fresh, crisp salad made from the ingredients listed, or those of your own choice. (Add dressing as desired.)

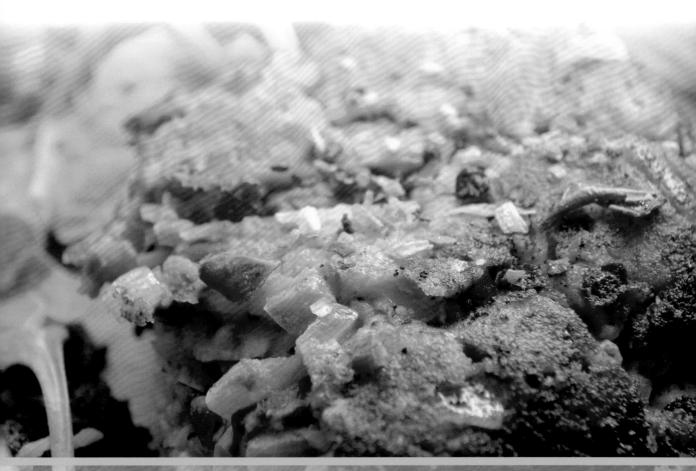

Spicy Rice with Vegetables

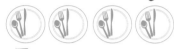

Ingredients

1 tsp olive oil
2 shallots, finely chopped
1 clove garlic, crushed
2 tsp garam masala
1 tsp turmeric
½ tsp ground cumin
10 oz / 280g / 1¼ cups brown rice
18 fl oz / 500mls vegetable stock or water
Salt and black pepper
4oz / 115g / ½ cup fresh or frozen peas
4oz / 115g / ½ cup fresh or frozen sweetcorn
3 tbsp fresh coriander (chopped)

Preparation Method

• In a saucepan that has a lid, sauté the shallots and garlic in the olive oil for about 5 minutes.

• Add the spices and the rice and stir thoroughly. Season with salt and pepper. Add the liquid and bring to the boil, then put the lid on, turn down the heat and cook for about 25 minutes.

• Add the peas and sweetcorn, replace the lid and cook for another 10 minutes. Remove from the heat and allow to stand for a further 5 minutes.

• Fluff up the rice with a fork and mix the peas and sweetcorn through. Serve in bowls, topped with the chopped coriander.

If you prefer, cook the dish in a covered casserole in the oven (at 200°C / 390°F / gas mark 6).

Spicy Vegetable Stew

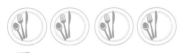 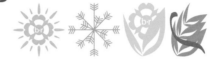

Ingredients

1 large onion, thinly sliced
3 garlic cloves, crushed
½ pint / 285mls vegetable stock
1 tbsp chilli powder (or to taste)
1 tsp ground coriander
1 large sweet potato, peeled and chopped
2 tins (15oz / 400g) chopped tomatoes
2 courgettes, finely diced
7oz / 200g / 1 cup baby spinach
4 tbsp chopped coriander

Preparation Method

• Dry fry the onion and garlic in a non-stick pan for 3-4 minutes, then pour in the stock and add the chilli powder, coriander and sweet potato. Bring to the boil and simmer for ten minutes

• Add the tomatoes and courgettes; bring back to the boil and simmer for another 10 minutes.

• Using a slotted spoon, fish out about half the sweet potato and mash it, then return to the stew and stir through (to thicken it slightly).

• Fold in the spinach so that it wilts into the pan.

• Serve in bowls, garnished with the chopped coriander

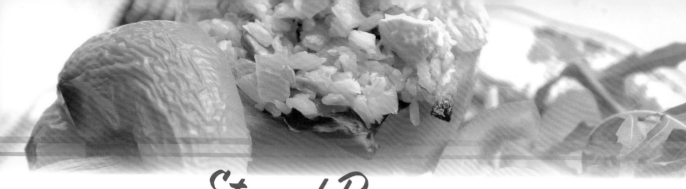

Stuffed Peppers with Salad

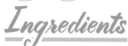

Ingredients

2 large red or yellow peppers
2 tbsps olive oil
1 large onion, chopped
2 cloves garlic, crushed
1 tbsp pine nuts
4oz / 115g / $\frac{1}{2}$ cup cooked brown rice
4oz / 115g / $\frac{1}{2}$ cup mushrooms, sliced
2oz / 55g / $\frac{1}{4}$ cup feta cheese
Fresh basil
Salt and freshly ground black pepper
FOR THE SALAD:
Rocket
Tomatoes
Spring onions
Radish
Pepper

Preparation Method

• Cut the tops off the peppers and set to one side. Remove the seeds and pith.
• Sauté the onions and garlic in about $\frac{3}{4}$ of the olive oil for 3-4 minutes. Add the mushrooms and cook for a further couple of minutes.
• Thoroughly combine all the ingredients in a bowl and use the mixture to stuff the peppers. Put the tops back on.
• Preheat the oven to 200°C / 390°F / gas mark 6, pace the peppers on a lightly oiled baking tray (use the remaining olive oil) and bake for 30-35 minutes.
• Serve with a fresh, crisp salad made from the ingredients listed, or those of your own choice. (Add dressing as desired.)

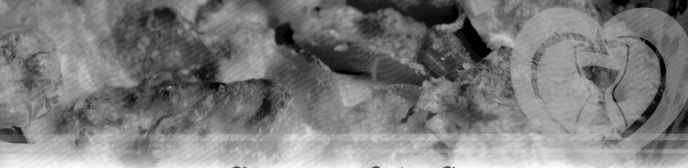

Summer Veg Gratin

Ingredients

3 tbsps olive oil
2 red onions, thinly sliced
2 cloves garlic, crushed
2 courgettes, sliced
2 yellow summer squash (or other summer squash), sliced
12oz / 340g / 1½ cups ripe tomatoes, sliced and placed on kitchen paper to absorb juices
4oz / 115g / ½ cup grated parmesan
4oz / 115g / ½ cup grated mozzarella
Large sprig of fresh basil, chopped
Salt and freshly ground black pepper

Preparation Method

• Heat 1 tbsp olive oil in a frying pan and sauté the onions, stirring frequently, for around 10 minutes. Add the garlic for the last couple of minutes.

• Lightly oil an ovenproof dish and spread the onions and garlic evenly in the bottom. Preheat the oven to 180°C / 350°F / gas mark 4.

• Put 1 tbsp oil in a bowl; add the sliced courgettes and squash and turn in the oil until coated.

• Mix the parmesan, mozzarella and basil together and set half aside. Layer the sliced vegetables over the onions in the dish, sprinkling each layer with the cheese mix. Top the final layer with the reserved cheese and season with salt and pepper.

• Bake for around an hour until well-browned. Allow to stand for 15 minutes before serving.

This is delicious on its own or with a crunchy salad. Alternatively, serve it with your favourite fish.

Sweet Potato, Lentil & Coconut Curry

Ingredients

2 large sweet potatoes (approx 3lbs / 1$\frac{1}{2}$kg / 6 cups)
20 black olives (or to your taste)
1lb / 500g / 2 cups of lentils
2 tins (400ml) of coconut milk
2 tins (15oz / 400g) chopped tomatoes
A handful of fresh coriander leaves
1 tbsp of turmeric
1 tbsp of cumin
1 tbsp of ground ginger
Salt and pepper
Juice of 1 lemon

Preparation Method

• Pre-heat the oven to 180°C / 350°F / gas mark 4.

• Cut the sweet potatoes into small bite-sized cubes and finely chop the coriander.

• Place the coconut milk, tomatoes, turmeric, cumin and ground ginger in a large saucepan (or even better, a Le Creuset style cast iron casserole dish). Allow ingredients to heat until they begin bubbling. At this point add the sweet potato cubes, lentils, olives and coriander, plus salt and pepper.

• Once everything is mixed, simply place the lid on the pot and place it in the oven to cook for about an hour, until the potatoes are soft and everything tastes delicious! At this point squeeze the lemon juice into the pot and then serve.

N.B. If you're making rice, simply put it on to boil while the pot is in the oven; time it so that the two finish cooking at the same time.

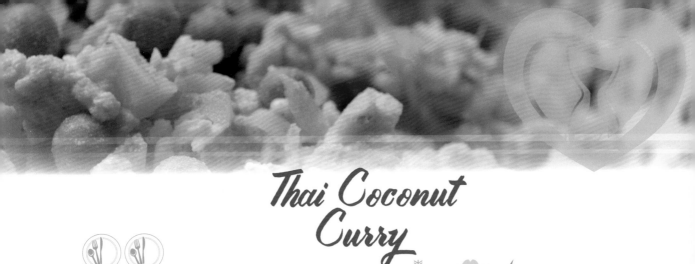

Thai Coconut Curry

Ingredients

1 tbsp coconut oil
2 cloves garlic, minced
½ onion, chopped
8oz / 225g / 1 cup firm tofu, cubed
1 tin (400ml) light coconut milk
½ pint / 285mls vegetable stock
2 stalks lemongrass, diced
½ red pepper, cut into strips
1 large carrot, cut into matchsticks
4oz / 115g / ½ cup peas, fresh or frozen
2 tbsp desiccated coconut
1 tbsp ground ginger
1 tbsps Thai red curry paste (or personal preference)
2-3 sprigs fresh basil leaves, chopped (reserve some leaves for a garnish)
6oz / 170g / ¾ cup brown rice

Preparation Method

• Sauté the garlic and onion in the oil for 2-3 minutes, then add the tofu and cook for a further 2-3 minutes.

• Add the coconut milk and vegetable stock and bring to the boil. Add the lemongrass, pepper, carrot, peas, desiccated coconut, ground ginger and curry paste. Reduce the heat and simmer for about 10 minutes until the vegetables are tender.

• Meanwhile cook the rice, timing it to be ready with the curry. Serve the rice in bowls with the curry spooned over the top; garnish with basil leaves.

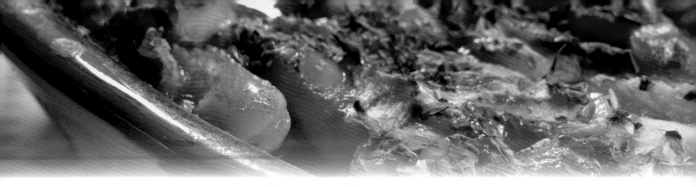

Three Bean Casserole

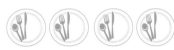

Ingredients

1 tin (15oz / 400g) red kidney beans, drained and rinsed
1 tin (15oz / 400g) cannellini beans, drained and rinsed
1 tin (15oz / 400g) borlotti beans, drained and rinsed
2 tins (15oz / 400g) chopped tomatoes
8oz / 225g / 1 cup chopped onion (frozen or pre-prepared)
8oz / 225g / 1 cup chopped mushrooms (frozen or pre-prepared)
1 tbsp mixed herbs

Preparation Method

• Preheat oven to 180°C / 350°F / gas mark 4.

• Put all ingredients into an ovenproof casserole dish and bake for an hour, or until vegetables are cooked.

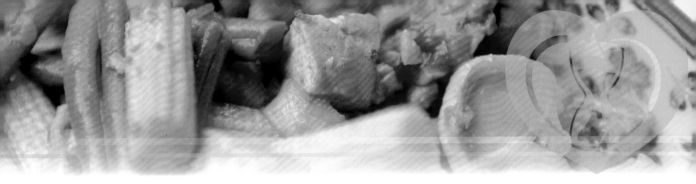

Tofu & Tomato Casserole

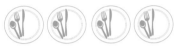

Ingredients

1 tin (15oz / 400g) chopped tomatoes
1 block tofu, diced
1 courgette, sliced
1 leek, chopped finely
1 tbsp dried mixed herbs
$1/2$ tsp chilli powder (optional)
12oz / 340g / $1^1/2$ cups green beans
12oz / 340g / $1^1/2$ cups baby sweetcorn, cut in half lengthways

Preparation Method

• Preheat the oven to 180°C / 350°F / gas mark 4.

• Put the chopped tomatoes, diced tofu, sliced courgette, chopped leek, dried herbs and chilli powder (if using) into an ovenproof casserole dish and put into the oven for around 30 minutes.

• Steam the green beans and baby sweetcorn, timing them to be ready when the casserole is cooked.

• Serve the casserole with the steamed veg on the side.

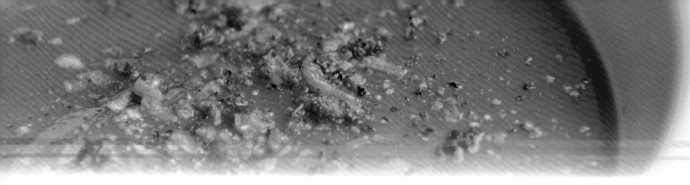

Tomato Soup

This is a delicious soup, simple and satisfying.

Ingredients

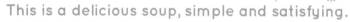

1 tsp olive oil
2 shallots, finely chopped
1 clove garlic, crushed
1 tin (15oz / 400g) chopped tomatoes
½ pint / 285mls vegetable stock or water
2 tsps smoked paprika
2-3 sprigs fresh basil
Salt and black pepper

Preparation Method

• Sauté the shallots and garlic in the olive oil for about 5 minutes.

• Add all other ingredients and stir thoroughly. Bring to the boil, stir, and simmer for about 15 minutes.

• Remove from heat and allow to cool slightly. Puree the soup until smooth.

• Reheat and add salt and pepper to taste.

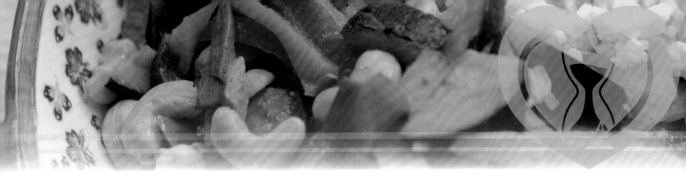

Traffic Light Stir Fry

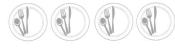

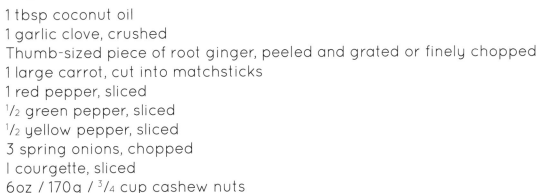

Ingredients

1 tbsp coconut oil
1 garlic clove, crushed
Thumb-sized piece of root ginger, peeled and grated or finely chopped
1 large carrot, cut into matchsticks
1 red pepper, sliced
$\frac{1}{2}$ green pepper, sliced
$\frac{1}{2}$ yellow pepper, sliced
3 spring onions, chopped
I courgette, sliced
6oz / 170g / $\frac{3}{4}$ cup cashew nuts
1 tbsp sesame oil

Preparation Method

• Heat the oil in a wok or frying pan. Add the garlic, ginger and carrot and stir fry for 1-2 minutes.

• Add the rest of the veg and stir fry for a further 3-4 minutes, then add the cashew nuts and stir fry for a further minute.

• Serve in bowls, drizzled with sesame oil.

Tuna & Mango Salsa

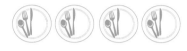 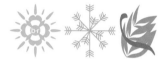

Ingredients

1 large mango, cut up into small cubes
$\frac{1}{2}$ red pepper, chopped
$\frac{1}{2}$ red onion, chopped
1 bunch chopped fresh coriander
2 tbsps rice vinegar
2 tbsps olive oil
4 x 6oz / 170g tuna steaks (about 1 inch thick)
Coconut oil

Preparation Method

* Mix all together all ingredients except the tuna and coconut oil. Season with salt and pepper.

* Rub the tuna steaks with the coconut oil and grill for 4 minutes on each side.

* Serve salsa on tuna steak.

Mango is rich in tartaric acid, malic acid and traces of citric acid that alkalise the body.

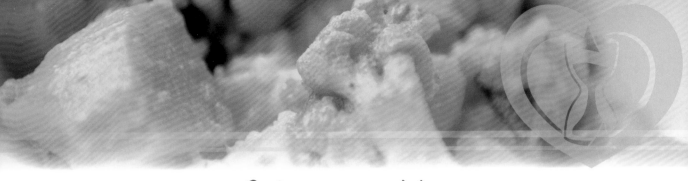

Vegetable Korma

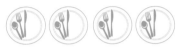

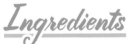

Ingredients

1 tbsp coconut oil
1 dried red chilli, minced
2 onions, finely chopped
1 tsp ground coriander
Pinch of ground black pepper
1 tsp turmeric
1 tsp garam masala
1 small cauliflower, separated into florets
2 carrots, cut into chunks
1 courgette, sliced
2 potatoes, peeled and cut into chunks
1 tin (400 ml) coconut milk
Fresh coriander, chopped
10 oz basmati rice

Preparation Method

• The curry will take around half an hour to cook, so put the rice on to cook, timing it to be ready at the same time.

• Heat the oil in a saucepan and sauté the onions for 5 minutes. Add the chilli and spices and cook for a further minute.

• Add the vegetables and cook for 2-3 minutes, stirring to ensure they are evenly coated with oil and spices.

• Add the coconut milk and cook for a further 10-15 minutes, until the vegetables are tender.

• Garnish with coriander and serve with the basmati rice.

Veggie Burgers & Sweet Potato Chips

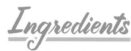

Ingredients

FOR THE CHIPS:
2 sweet potatoes, scrubbed and cut into large chips
1 tbsp olive oil
Freshly ground black pepper
1 tsp smoked paprika (optional)
FOR THE BURGERS:
1 tin (15oz / 400g) chickpeas (garbanzo beans) rinsed
1 small carrot, grated
$^1/_2$ red onion, sliced
1 tsp lemon juice
$3^1/_2$oz / 100g / 0.4 cup ground almonds
1 tsp ground cumin
1 tbsp fresh coriander, chopped
1 egg
Brown rice flour

Preparation Method

• Preheat the oven to 200°C / 390°F / gas mark 6 and line a baking tray with parchment paper.

• In a large bowl, toss the sweet potato chips with the oil. Transfer to the baking tray and season with black pepper and smoked paprika, if using. Bake for around 35 minutes, turning occasionally.

• Meanwhile, put all the ingredients for the burgers, apart from the egg

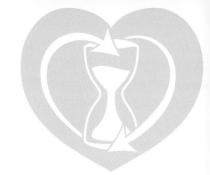

and the flour, in a food processor and process to the consistency of breadcrumbs. Add the egg and pulse to mix it in.

• With floured hands, shape the mixture into four patties. Flour the patties, then place on a baking tray covered in baking parchment. Put into the oven with the chips for the last 15-20 minutes of cooking time.

• Serve the burgers and chips with a nice, crisp salad.

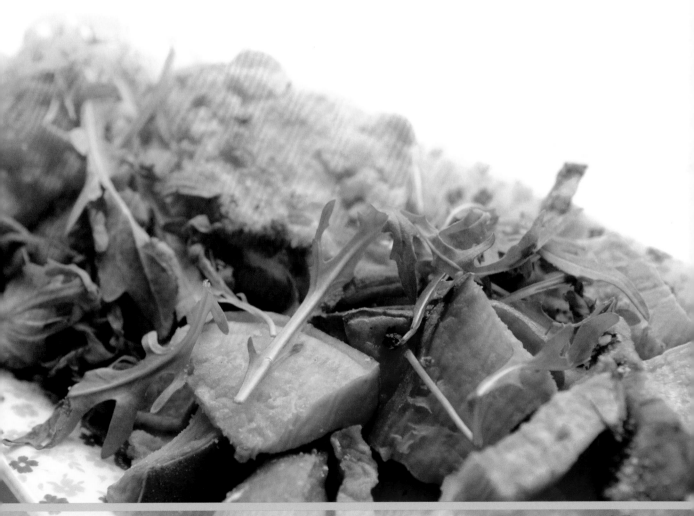

CHAPTER 7

Shopping Lists

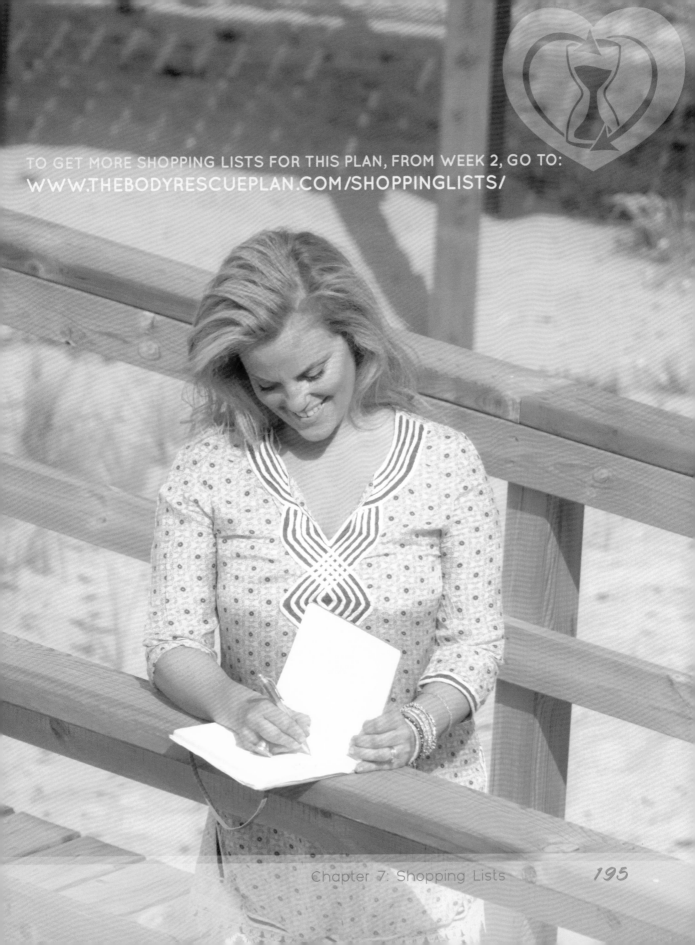

TO GET MORE SHOPPING LISTS FOR THIS PLAN, FROM WEEK 2, GO TO:
WWW.THEBODYRESCUEPLAN.COM/SHOPPINGLISTS/

FRESH VEGETABLES
- 4 sweet potatoes
- 4 portobello mushrooms
- 1 punnet chestnut mushrooms
- 1 punnet mushrooms
- 1 aubergine
- 2 large avocados
- 1 small onion
- 3 large onions
- 1 red onion
- 3 large red peppers
- 3 green peppers
- 2 yellow peppers
- 1 butternut squash
- 1 fresh beetroot
- 1 pack (10^1/₂oz / 300g) ready-cooked vacuum packed beetroot
- 1 tray baby corn
- 1 tray green beans
- 1 bag mung bean sprouts
- 2 cucumbers
- 1 head celery
- 1 handful of kale
- 8 carrots
- 1 punnet cherry tomatoes
- 5 beef tomatoes
- 2 trays salad tomatoes
- 1 head romaine lettuce
- 1 bag spinach
- 5 bags rocket
- 1 bunch radishes
- 2 bunches spring onions
- 1lb / 500g peas
- 1 small courgette
- 1 bulb garlic

FRESH FRUIT
- 7 apples
- 1 ripe mango
- 4 ripe bananas
- 1 orange
- 6 lemons
- 2 limes
- 4 fresh figs
- 10 dates
- 8oz / 225g dates
- 1^1/₂lbs / 700g fresh strawberries
- 4oz / 115g seedless grapes

DRIED FRUIT
- 2 packets raisins
- 1 packet dried apricots
- 1 packet sultanas
- 1 packet dried figs

FISH & SHELLFISH
- 1 tin mackerel in curry sauce
- 3^1/₂oz / 100g smoked salmon slices
- 12oz / 55g cooked peeled prawns
- 1 large tin (418g) wild red salmon

CARBS
- 2lbs / 1kg quinoa
- 1^1/₄oz / 45g popped quinoa
- 1 bag oats
- 1 large packet pasta
- 4oz / 115g couscous
- 1 bag brown rice

NUTS & SEEDS
- 1 packet ground almonds
- Flaxseeds
- Chia seeds
- Sunflower seeds
- 2oz / 55g walnuts
- 2oz / 55g pecans

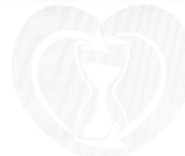

- 4oz / 115g almonds
- 4oz / 115g cashew nuts
- 4oz / 115g pistachios
- Pine nuts
- 1 packet flaked almonds

DRIED HERBS & SPICES
- Chilli flakes
- Chilli powder
- Paprika
- Smoked paprika
- Ground cardamom
- Mint
- Oregano
- Cinnamon
- Nutmeg
- Mixed spice
- Mustard seeds

FRESH HERBS & SPICES
- Parsley
- Flat-leaved parsley
- Mint
- Basil
- Coriander
- Chives
- Root ginger
- 1-2 fresh green chillies
- Jalapeno peppers

OTHER
- Dijon mustard
- Olive oil
- Coconut oil
- Toasted sesame oil
- Apple cider vinegar
- Balsamic vinegar
- Honey

- Maple syrup
- Vegetable stock / cubes
- Baking soda
- 1 large carton Greek yogurt
- 1 carton natural yogurt
- 1 large pot live yogurt
- 4$\frac{1}{2}$oz / 128g fromage frais
- 4oz / 115g soft goat's cheese
- Maca powder
- Vanilla extract
- Raw cacao powder
- Rice flour
- 1 tub hummus
- 1 tin (15oz / 400g) green lentils
- 1 tin (15oz / 400g) red kidney beans
- 1 tin (15oz / 400g) cannellini beans
- 1 jar tahini
- 1 jar capers
- $\frac{2}{3}$ pint / 350mls rice milk
- $\frac{1}{4}$ pint / 150mls almond milk
- 2oz / 55g unsweetened almond milk
- 1 tin (400ml) coconut milk
- 12$\frac{1}{2}$oz / 350g feta cheese
- 6oz / 170g goat's cheese
- 1 carton cream cheese
- 8 eggs
- 1 tub almond butter
- 1 nori sheet
- 1 carton apple juice
- 1 carton orange juice
- 1 bottle light soy sauce
- 1 bottle sweet chilli sauce (no added sugar, e.g. Trinity Hill Farms)
- 1 tube tomato puree
- 8oz / 225g smoked tofu, cubed
- Himalayan salt
- Black pepper
- Small cake cases

SHOPPING LISTS
Winter
WEEK 1

FRESH VEGETABLES
- 8 sweet potatoes
- 2 celeriac
- 1 sweetcorn cob
- 1 jacket potato
- 3 large potatoes
- 1 cauliflower
- 4 portobello mushrooms
- 2 punnets chestnut mushrooms
- 1 aubergine
- 2 large avocados
- 1 small onion
- 3 large onions
- 4 red onions
- 6 red peppers
- 2 green peppers
- 3 yellow peppers
- 1 butternut squash
- 4 fresh beetroot
- 1 tray baby corn
- 1 tray green beans
- 2 cucumbers
- 1 head celery
- 1 large bunch kale
- 4 carrots
- 2 punnets cherry tomatoes
- 1 punnet mixed tomatoes
- 1 beef tomatoes
- 1 tray salad tomatoes
- 2 heads romaine lettuce
- 2 bags spinach
- 4 bags rocket
- 1 bunch radishes
- 2 bunches spring onions
- 1lb / 500g peas
- 5 courgettes
- 2 bulbs garlic

FRESH FRUIT

- 1lb / 500g plantains / green bananas
- 1 banana
- Punnet raspberries
- Punnet blackberries
- 6 apples
- 1 ripe mango
- 1 orange
- 6 lemons
- 2 limes
- 2 fresh figs
- 10 dates
- 4oz / 115g dates

DRIED FRUIT
- 2 packets raisins
- 1 packet dried apricots
- 1 packet dried figs

FISH & SHELLFISH
- 10$\frac{1}{2}$oz / 300g smoked salmon
- 1 tin anchovies
- 1 tin tuna

CARBS
- 1lb / 454g quinoa
- 1$\frac{1}{4}$oz / 45g popped quinoa
- 1 bag oats
- 2$\frac{1}{2}$oz / 75g organic puffed rice (e.g. Kallo)
- 1 bag brown rice
- 8oz / 225g Arborio rice

NUTS & SEEDS
- 1 packet ground almonds
- Flaxseeds
- Chia seeds
- Sesame seeds
- Sunflower seeds

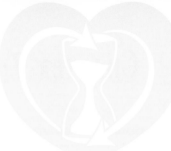

- 2oz / 55g walnuts
- 2oz / 55g pecans
- 4oz / 115g almonds
- 10oz / 285g cashew nuts
- 4oz / 115g pistachios
- Pine nuts

DRIED HERBS & SPICES
- Chilli powder
- Paprika
- Smoked paprika
- Ground cardamom
- Ground coriander
- Ground cumin
- Curry powder
- Turmeric
- Cayenne pepper
- Dried mixed herbs
- Rosemary
- Cinnamon
- Ground ginger
- Nutmeg
- Mixed spice

FRESH HERBS & SPICES
- Parsley
- Basil
- Coriander
- Root ginger
- 1-2 fresh green chillies

OTHER
- Olive oil
- Coconut oil
- Toasted sesame oil
- Sesame oil
- Apple cider vinegar
- Balsamic vinegar

- Honey
- Maple syrup
- Rice syrup
- Vegetable stock / cubes
- 1 tub low fat Greek yogurt
- 1 carton natural yogurt
- 1 large carton fromage frais
- Maca powder
- 1 vanilla pod
- Vanilla extract
- Raw cacao powder
- Cornflour
- Brown rice flour
- 1lb / 500g lentils
- 5$\frac{1}{2}$oz / 150g creamed coconut
- 2 tins (400ml) coconut milk
- 2 tins (15oz / 400g) chickpeas
- 1 tin (15oz / 400g) red kidney beans
- 2 tins (15oz / 400g) tinned tomatoes
- 3 tins(15oz/400g)chopped tomatoes
- 1 jar tahini
- 2 jars black olives
- 2.75 pints / 1.6 litres almond milk
- $\frac{1}{4}$ pint / 140ml soya milk
- 2oz / 55g cheddar cheese
- 7 eggs
- 1 tub almond butter
- 1 carton apple juice
- 1 carton orange juice
- 1 bottle light soy sauce
- 1 bottle sweet chilli sauce
- 1 tube tomato puree
- 8oz / 225g smoked tofu, cubed
- 1 loaf rye bread
- Coarse sea salt
- Himalayan salt
- Black pepper
- Small cake cases

FRESH VEGETABLES

- 5 sweet potatoes
- 2 large potatoes
- 2lbs / 1kg potatoes
- 4 portobello mushrooms
- 1 punnet chestnut mushrooms
- 1 punnet mushrooms
- 1 aubergine
- 1 large avocado
- 1 small onion
- 4 large onions
- 5 red peppers
- 1 green pepper
- 2 yellow peppers
- 1 butternut squash
- 3 fresh beetroot
- 1 pack (10$\frac{1}{2}$oz / 300g) ready-cooked vacuum packed beetroots
- 3 cucumbers
- 2 heads celery
- 1 large bunch kale
- 4 carrots
- 2 parsnips
- 2 punnets cherry tomatoes
- 1 tray salad tomatoes
- 5 bags rocket
- 1 bunch radishes
- 1 bunch spring onions
- 4 courgettes
- 2 bulbs garlic

FRESH FRUIT

- 1lb / 500g plantains / green bananas
- Punnet raspberries
- 8oz / 225g açaí berries
- 2 apples
- 1 ripe mango
- 5 bananas
- 1$\frac{1}{2}$lbs / 700g fresh strawberries
- 1 orange
- 4 lemons
- 1 lime
- 5$\frac{1}{2}$oz / 150g Medjool dates
- 3 whole Medjool dates
- 10 dates
- 4oz / 115g seedless grapes

DRIED FRUIT

- 1 packet raisins
- 9oz / 250g dried mixed fruit

CARBS

- 1 bag oats
- 4oz / 115g couscous
- 2$\frac{1}{2}$oz / 75g organic puffed rice (e.g. Kallo)
- 1 bag puffed brown rice
- 1 bag brown rice
- 1 packet Biona Organic Rice Cakes with Quinoa

NUTS & SEEDS

- 1 packet ground almonds
- Flaxseeds
- Chia seeds
- Sesame seeds
- Sunflower seeds
- 1 packet flaked almonds
- 6oz / 170g cashew nuts
- 3$\frac{1}{2}$oz / 100g mixed nuts
- 8oz / 225g pistachio nuts
- Pine nuts

DRIED HERBS & SPICES

- Chilli flakes
- Chilli powder

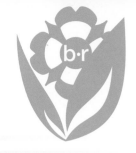
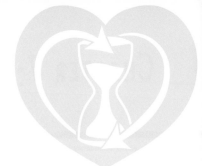

- Paprika
- Smoked paprika
- Ground cardamom
- Ground coriander
- Ground cumin
- Turmeric
- Cayenne pepper
- Bouquet garni
- Dried mixed herbs
- Cinnamon
- Ground ginger
- Nutmeg
- Mint

FRESH HERBS & SPICES
- Flat-leaved parsley
- Dill
- Basil
- Mint
- Coriander
- Root ginger
- 1-2 fresh green chillies

OTHER
- Dijon mustard
- Olive oil
- Coconut oil
- Sesame oil
- Apple cider vinegar
- Honey
- Maple syrup
- Rice syrup
- Vegetable stock / cubes
- 2 large tubs Greek yogurt
- 2 cartons natural yogurt
- 1 large carton fromage frais
- Maca powder
- 3$\frac{1}{2}$ oz / 100g almond powder

- Vanilla extract
- Raw cacao powder
- Baking soda
- Cornflour
- 1lb / 500g lentils
- 5$\frac{1}{2}$oz / 150g creamed coconut
- 4 large cans of coconut milk
- Large can cooked green lentils
- 1 tin (15oz / 400g) chickpeas
- 2 tins (15oz / 400g) tinned tomatoes
- 3 tins(15oz/400g)chopped tomatoes
- 2 jars black olives
- 1 jar piquant red peppers (e.g. Pep-padew)
- 1 tub soft cheese
- Coconut flakes
- $\frac{1}{4}$ pint / 150mls almond milk
- 4fl oz / 120mls unsweetened almond milk
- 2oz / 60g unsweetened almond milk
- $\frac{2}{3}$ pint / 350mls rice milk
- $\frac{1}{4}$ pint / 140mls soya milk
- 1 tub cashew nut butter
- 12$\frac{1}{2}$oz / 355g feta cheese
- 6oz / 170g goat's cheese
- 14 eggs
- 1 loaf rye bread
- Coarse sea salt
- Himalayan salt
- Black pepper

FRESH VEGETABLES

- 8 sweet potatoes
- 4 portobello mushrooms
- 1 punnet chestnut mushrooms
- 1 punnet mushrooms
- 1 aubergine
- 1 avocado
- 1 red onion
- 3 large red peppers
- 2 green peppers
- 1 yellow pepper
- 2 cauliflowers
- 2 celeriac
- 2¼lbs / 1kg Jap pumpkin
- 4 fresh beetroot
- 1 tray baby corn
- 2 trays green beans
- 1 cucumber
- 2 heads celery
- 2 bunches asparagus
- 1 bag spinach
- 1 bag kale
- 10 carrots
- 1 small pak choi
- 2 punnets cherry tomatoes
- 1 tray salad tomatoes
- 5 bags rocket
- 1 bunch radishes
- 1 bunch spring onions
- 1lb / 500g peas
- 3 courgettes
- 2 bulbs garlic

FRESH FRUIT

- 7 apples
- 1 ripe mango
- 7 bananas
- 1lb / 500g plantains / green bananas

- 4oz / 115g blueberries
- 1 punnet raspberries
- 1 punnet blackberries
- 6 lemons
- 3 limes
- 2 fresh figs
- 7 dates
- 3½oz / 90g dates
- 3 whole Medjool dates
- 1½lbs / 700g fresh strawberries
- 1lb / 500g grapes
- 4oz / 115g seedless grapes

DRIED FRUIT

- 2 packets raisins
- 1 packet sultanas
- 1 packet dried figs
- 1 packet mixed dried fruit

FISH & SHELLFISH

- 8oz / 225g smoked haddock fillets
- 10½oz / 300g smoked salmon
- 8oz / 225g uncooked prawns
- 1 tin anchovies

CARBS

- 5½oz / 150g buckwheat
- 8oz / 225g quinoa
- 1 large bag oats
- 8oz / 225g / Arborio rice
- 1 bag basmati rice
- 1 bag brown rice

NUTS & SEEDS

- 1 packet ground almonds
- Flaxseeds
- Chia seeds
- Sesame seeds

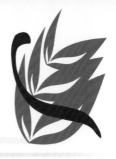
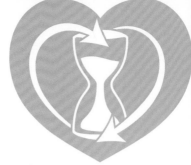

- Sunflower seeds
- 3½oz / 100g mixed nuts
- 2oz / 55g walnuts
- 2oz / 55g pecans
- 2½oz / 75g roasted pistachios
- Pine nuts

DRIED HERBS & SPICES
- Medium curry powder
- Turmeric
- Ground cumin
- Ground ginger
- Garlic powder
- Rosemary
- Cinnamon
- Mixed spice
- Dried mixed herbs

FRESH HERBS & SPICES
- Parsley
- Mint
- Basil
- Coriander
- Root ginger
- 1 vanilla pod
- 1 red chilli
- 1 stalk lemongrass

OTHER
- Olive oil
- Coconut oil
- Toasted sesame oil
- Apple cider vinegar
- Honey
- Maple syrup
- Vegetable stock / cubes
- 1 carton Greek yogurt
- 1 large pot natural yogurt

- 1 large pot live yogurt
- 1 pot fromage frais
- 1 tub cashew nut butter
- Coconut flakes
- Vanilla extract
- Raw cacao powder
- Cornflour
- Brown rice flour
- Buckwheat flour
- 1 tub hummus
- 1 tin (15oz / 400g) chickpeas
- 1 tin (15oz / 400g) chopped tomatoes
- 1 jar black olives
- 1 jar tahini
- ⅔ pint / 350mls rice milk
- 2oz / 55g unsweetened almond milk
- 3 pints / 1.75 litres almond milk
- ¼ pint / 140mls soya milk
- 1 tin (400ml) coconut milk
- 10oz / 280g feta cheese
- 10 eggs
- 1 tub almond butter
- 1 carton apple juice
- 1 carton orange juice
- 1 bottle fish sauce
- 1 bottle light soy sauce
- 1 bottle sweet chilli sauce (no added sugar, e.g. Trinity Hill Farms)
- 1 tube tomato puree
- 8oz / 225g smoked tofu, cubed
- Coarse sea salt
- Himalayan salt
- Black pepper

CHAPTER 8

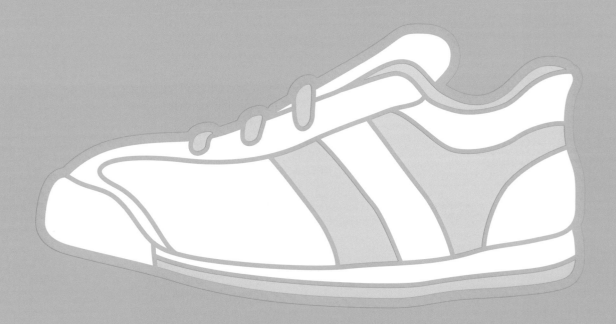

Exercises

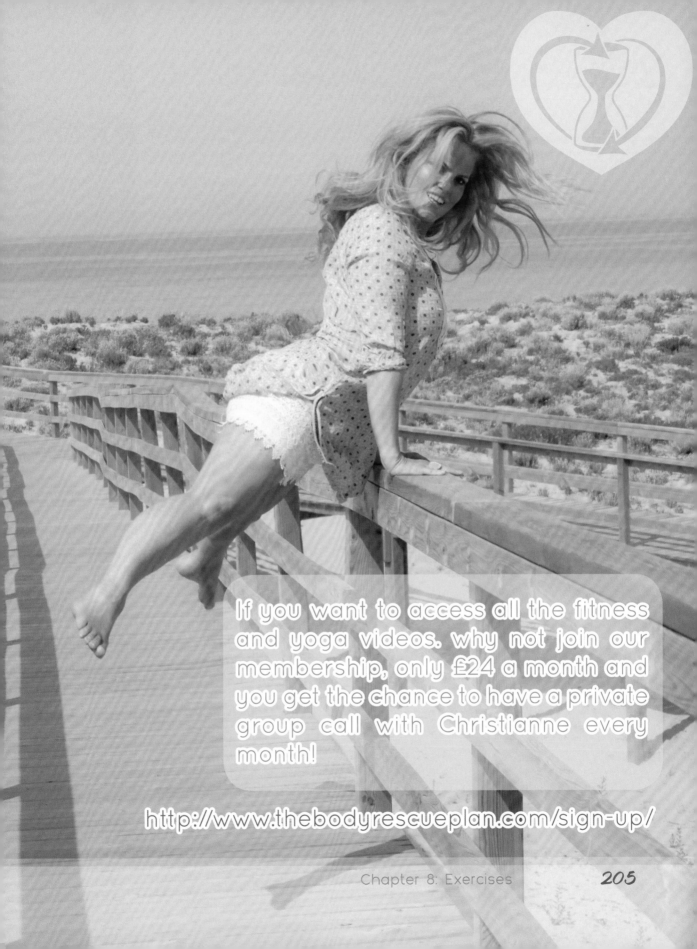

If you want to access all the fitness and yoga videos. why not join our membership, only £24 a month and you get the chance to have a private group call with Christianne every month!

http://www.thebodyrescueplan.com/sign-up/

CHAPTER 8: *Exercises*

The maintenance plan exercise programme follows the same format as The Body Rescue Plan. Again, I want to make this as simple as possible for you. You have done the groundwork in the first twelve weeks, so now this wants to feel like part of your life, as much part of your routine as brushing your teeth. To stop you getting bored I have added lots more varied exercises within the sections, with the exception of the warm up and the stretch, which I have kept the same so you can just enjoy and relax with them. I have developed a new plan for you in the Yoga section, with the mindset to increase each posture over time.

These are developed into a six month plan for you, so you will never get bored and can then sustain or increase your fitness. After the six month period I teach you how to adapt these exercises, to add new plans for yourself, or you can swap and change the plans you have already used.

The exercises are:

Interval 3, Resistance 3, Yoga, Cardio and Abs 3 – for the first two months.
Interval 4, Resistance 4, Yoga, Cardio and Abs 4 – for months three and four.
Interval 5, Resistance 5, Yoga, Cardio and Abs 5 – for months five and six.

Rules of Exercise

Do Resistance once a week, Interval once a week, Cardio three times a week, Yoga once a week and Abs every day. Always have one day off a week. You may rearrange this plan depending on your diary; for instance, you may want to do a lot of your workouts at the weekend – I have just written Sunday as a day off for ease, but if you want a day off in the week that is fine. Just don't do Interval and Resistance training on two consecutive days.

ALWAYS WARM UP AT THE START AND COOL DOWN AT THE END, WITH A STRETCH!

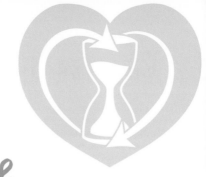

Warm up & Stretch

Go through each joint and roll in both directions for about 30 seconds on each joint. Then start warming up by marching on the spot, taking your arms in the air and circling them around you. After 3 minutes do a light jog, if you are able, until you are warm – around 7 minutes.

Hamstring Stretch on Back

Lie on your back and raise your right leg in the air; your left knee should be bent, with the foot on the floor. Put your hands behind your right leg and pull it towards you.
HOLD FOR 10 SECONDS. REPEAT WITH THE LEFT LEG.

Hip Stretch on Back

In the same position, place your right foot on your left thigh, and your hands behind your left leg. Keep your head on the floor. Raise your left foot off the floor, bringing the leg towards you.
HOLD FOR 10 SECONDS.

Forward Bend

In a seated position, straighten your legs in front of you, together. Reach to your feet.
HOLD FOR 10 SECONDS.

Seated Butterfly

In a seated position, place your feet together, knees out to the side, and try and push your knees to the floor.
HOLD FOR 10 SECONDS.

CHAPTER 8: Exercises

Seated Wide Leg

Take your legs wide and lean forwards, towards the floor.
HOLD FOR 20 SECONDS.

Child's Pose

From a kneeling position, take your head to the floor in front of you. Take your hands round towards your feet – hold your ankles if you can. You can make this easier by widening the legs.
HOLD FOR 10 SECONDS.

Standing Quad Stretch

Stand and hold onto your right foot, with your right hand, knee touching the other knee.
HOLD 10 SECONDS. REPEAT OTHER SIDE.

Shoulder Stretch

Take your right arm across your chest, towards your left shoulder. Take your left hand and pull onto the right forearm towards you.
HOLD 10 SECONDS. REPEAT OTHER SIDE.

Lower Back Stretch

Hug your right knee towards you, and straighten the left leg on the floor. Take your right arm out to the side and roll the hip to the left.
HOLD FOR 10 SECONDS. REPEAT OTHER SIDE.

Tricep Stretch

Take your right arm up in the air, bend it at the elbow and place your right

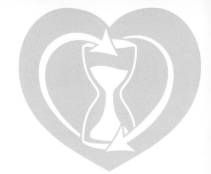

hand on the back of your neck. Reach your left arm up your back to find your right hand and clasp them together if you can. If you cannot make them meet, a good tip is to hold on to a sock with the upper hand, let it dangle and grab it with the lower hand, then walk the hands together. HOLD FOR 10 SECONDS. DO RIGHT AND LEFT.

Calf Stretch

Place your hands on the wall. Take your right leg back and push through the heel, feeling a deep calf stretch, bending the left leg, too. HOLD FOR 10 SECONDS. REPEAT OTHER SIDE.

Chest Stretch

Place your hands in the arch of your back, palms down. Squeeze your elbows in towards each other. If you can, get someone else to gently push your elbows together. This feels amazing, as most of the day we are rounded in the back, driving, texting, typing, etc. HOLD FOR 20 SECONDS.

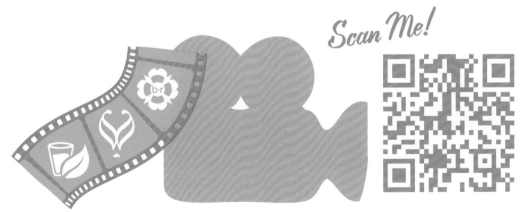

Watch our video for warm up and stretches here:

www.thebodyrescueplan.com/warmup/

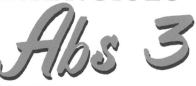

DO EVERYDAY

Head Rest Sit-up

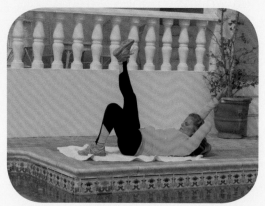

Lie on your back, bend your knees and place your feet on the floor. Take your left arm behind your head and straighten your right arm. If you can, hold onto your right arm with your left hand. Keeping your right arm by your right ear, lift your head and shoulders off the floor and breathe out. At the same time raise your left leg, and lean your right hand towards your left foot. Lower yourself back down and breathe out. Complete the set and repeat the other side.

Isometric Scissor

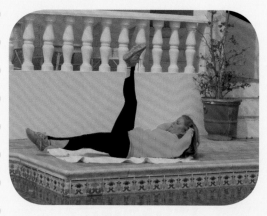

Lie on your back and lift your right leg, bringing it towards you. Keep it straight. Hold onto your right leg with both hands. Straighten your left leg in front of you. If you can, place your hands either side of your head. If that is too difficult, just hold onto your leg.

In this held position, breathe and focus on pulling your abs in. If your back feels uncomfortable you can bend your knees a little; alternatively, don't lower the left leg down so far. Do the set of breaths and then repeat to the other side.

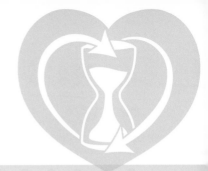

Twist Kick Thrust

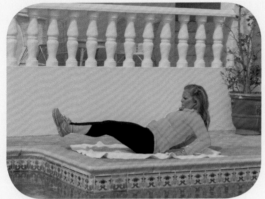

Sit down and place your hands on the floor, with your fingers forward.

Take your feet off the floor and bend your knees, pulling your knees towards your chest. As you do this, lean over to your right hip and stretch your legs out, then pull your knees in towards you again, lean over on your left hip, and stretch your legs out.

When you do this, straighten your legs as much as you can. Keep repeating.

Frog Sit-up

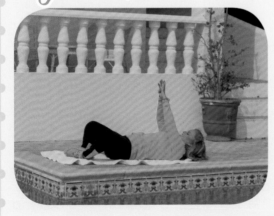

Lie on your back, bend your knees and touch the soles of your feet together, knees flopped out either side of you.

Stretch your arms behind you, then lift your head and shoulders off the floor and reach your hands towards your feet, breathing out.

Lower back down again and repeat.

Scissor Dance

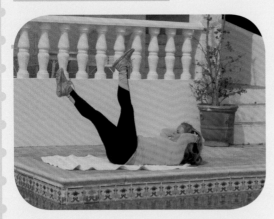

Lie on your back with your hands either side of your head. Raise both of your legs up to the ceiling and lift your head and shoulders off the floor.

Breathing out, lower your left leg to the floor. Breathe in. Then breathing out, lower your right leg down to meet your left leg so they are both stretched out in front of you. (If this causes too much tension on your back, bend your knees or don't lower your legs down as far.)

Then breathe in and raise first your right leg and then your left leg. And repeat. Do the set and then start on the other side.

Twisting Lean Backs

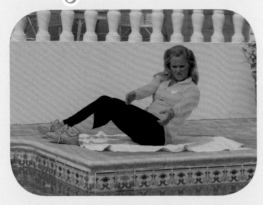

Sit down and bend your knees, your feet on the floor. Stretch your arms out in front of you, hands together.

Twist your whole body, keeping your arms in front of you, then lean back a bit, breathing out.

Sit up a little (but not all the way up), breathe in, twist to the other side and lean back again.

Do this 6 times and then come all the way up. And then do the set again.

	Head Rest Sit-up	Isometric Scissor	Twist Kick Thrust	Frog Sit-up	Scissor Dance	Twisting Lean Backs
Week 1	8 right & left	5 breaths right & left	6	9	4 right & left	twist for 4, do 1 time
Week 2	8 right & left	6 breaths right & left	6	10	5 right & left	twist for 6, do 1 time
Week 3	9 right & left	6 breaths right & left	6	11	6 right & left	twist for 6, do 1 time
Week 4	10 right & left	7 breaths right & left	8	12	6 right & left	twist for 4, do 2 times
Week 5	11 right & left	7 breaths right & left	8	13	7 right & left	twist for 4, do 2 times
Week 6	13 right & left	8 breaths right & left	8	14	8 right & left	twist for 6, do 2 times
Week 7	14 right & left	9 breaths right & left	10	15	9 right & left	twist for 4, do 3 times
Week 8	15 right & left	10 breaths right & left	12	16	10 right & left	twist for 6, do 3 times

Extended Bridge — BRIDGE LIFTS, 2 SETS OF 20

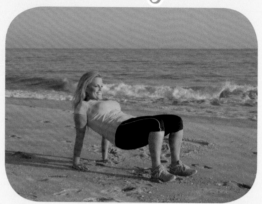

Sit down with your knees bent and your feet flat on the floor. Put your hands on the floor with your fingers forward.

Lift your hips off the floor, keeping your arms straight and pushing through your heels. Lower down slowly and repeat.

Runner's Plank — 2 SETS OF 16

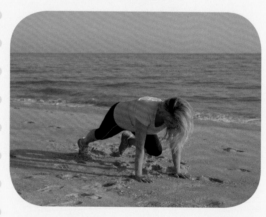

Start in an extended plank position, hands and balls of feet on the floor, body straight and fingers forward.

Take your right knee towards your right elbow, controlled and slow. Keep your shoulders steady. Take your right foot back again and repeat other side.

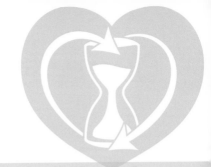

Stuck in the Mud Lunge – PUNCH 30 TIMES

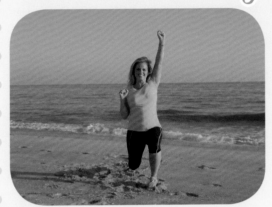

Go to a lunge position with your right foot behind you, your right knee bending towards the floor.

Hold in this position and punch to the ceiling, fast. Repeat other leg.

Sliding Lunge – RIGHT & LEFT, 15 TIMES

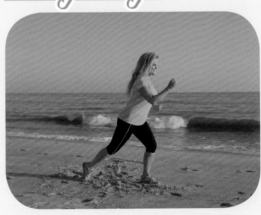

You need something that slides for this exercise, so get a towel or sock for a wooden floor, or use a plastic plate for a carpeted floor.

Put the ball of your right foot on the sock / plate and slide it back behind you, keeping your body upright. Take your right knee towards the floor, making sure your left knee (or front knee) is in line with your ankle; slide back up again.

Continue until you've completed 15 sliding lunges on that side, then repeat with the left leg.

Resistance 3

The Lizard Press up - X 10

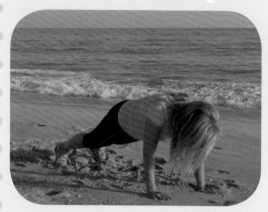

From a standing position, bend at the waist and place your hands on the floor. Walk your hands forward, trying to keep your hips still. As you get to an extended plank position, keep your elbows in and bend them towards your waist.

Straighten them again and then walk your hands back, again keeping your hips still. Repeat.

Lunge Twist - 2 SETS OF 12, RIGHT & LEFT

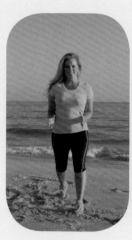 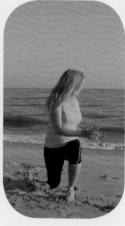

Stand in a lunge position, with your right leg behind you.

Take your hands out in front of you as if you are holding a ball and twist your body towards the left, making sure your eyes turn with your body.

Do a set and repeat the other side.

Interval 3

DO EACH EXERCISE FOR 20 SECONDS, THEN HAVE A 10 SECOND REST. ALL 8 EXERCISES EQUAL 1 ROUND; DO 4 ROUNDS

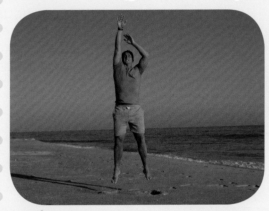

Squat to Shoot

From a squat position, jump up in the air as if you are shooting a ball through a hoop, and then back down, and repeat.

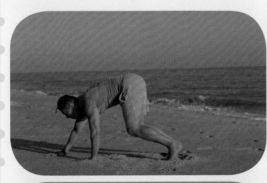

The Lion Plank

From a standing position, bend at the waist and walk your hands forward until you form an extended plank.

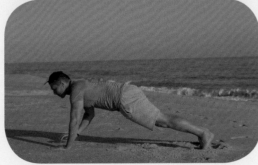

Next, drop to a normal plank, allowing your forearms to rest on the floor.

Finally raise yourself up again, placing your hands on the floor, and walk your hands back to your feet.

Repeat, trying to keep your hips as still as possible

EXERCISES
Interval 3

Morris Dancer

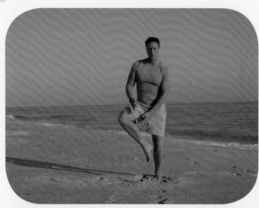

Jog on the spot, touching your right knee with your left hand and then your left knee with your right hand, and then your right ankle with your left hand and your left ankle with your right hand.

Plank Swing

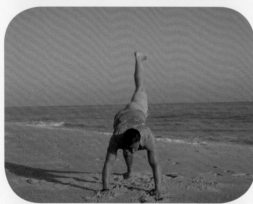

From an extended plank position, bring your right knee towards your right elbow and then back again. On round two do the other leg.

Twisted Sister Jacks

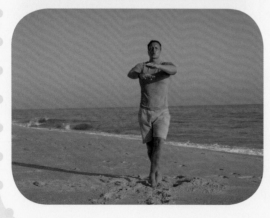

Stand with your feet together and arms by your sides. Jump, moving your feet apart and opening your arms. Jump again, this time crossing your feet and your arms. Jump again, landing with feet apart and arms wide. Jump again, this time crossing your feet and your arms the opposite way. Keep repeating.

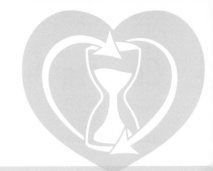

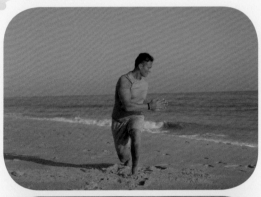

The Ooooh Lunge

Go into a lunge position: step your left foot forward and bend your right knee to the floor. Keep your left knee in line with your left ankle. Imagine you're holding on to a ball, and twist round to the left and then face the front and step back again. Repeat on the same leg, and then on round 2 do the other side.

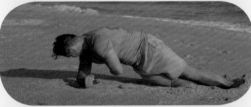

Mermaid Plank

Lie on your right side with your right elbow on the floor. Take your left foot over your right leg. Lift your hip off the floor and raise your left arm up in the air.
Now move your left hand under your right side and then back up again. If this is too difficult, just raise and lower without moving your arm.

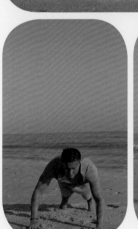
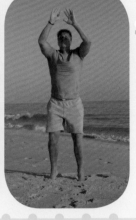

Press to Shoot

In a standing position, take your hands to the floor. Walk your hands forward and go to a press up position. Do one press up. Walk your hands back to your feet, trying to keep your hips still, then spring up and leap into the air.

EXERCISES
Yoga

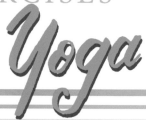

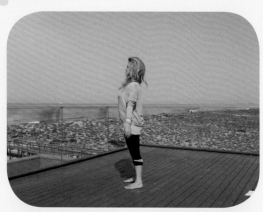

Mountain Pose – 5-10 BREATHS

Stand in the mountain pose and feel your feet connected to the earth. Find your position by rocking back and forth, first on your toes and then on your heels, then be balanced in the middle. Pull your shoulder blades down your back and focus on your breathing. Feel the breath expanding your ribcage.

Sun Salutation A

– DO THIS 3-5 TIMES

1 Take a deep breath in and stretch your arms up to the ceiling. Look to your hands.

2 Breathe out and take your arms to the floor. Look to your toes.

3 Look up and breathe in. Breath out and step back.

4 Take your knees to the floor. Press down, with your elbows in, chest leading, still breathing out. Look up and breathe in, taking your thighs off the floor but keeping the tops of your feet on the floor. If this is too much of a stretch for you, bend your elbows and keep thighs on the floor.

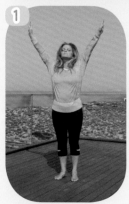
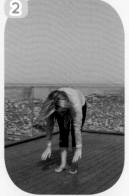
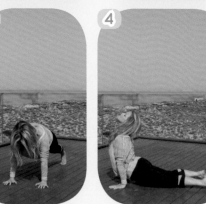

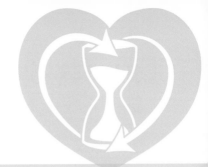

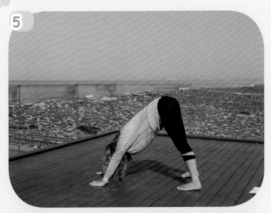

5 Breathe out, and round your back.

Take your knees off the floor and go to Downward Dog. Hold here for 5 breaths, pushing your heels into the floor and lifting your tail bone up to the ceiling. Open your shoulders, hands flat, thighs pulled up away from knees, chest pushed into the floor. Look to your knees.

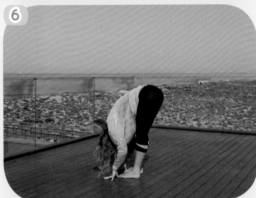

6 Step forward, putting your feet between your hands.

7 Look up; breathe in.

Look down; breathe out.

8 Stand up and breathe in, taking arms up to the ceiling.

Take arms to the side and assume Mountain Pose.

Take your arms to the floor and swing round left, then right, a few times.

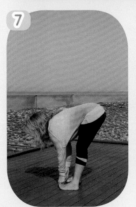
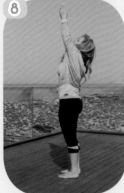

CHAPTER 8:

EXERCISES
Yoga
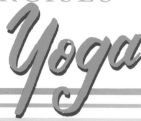

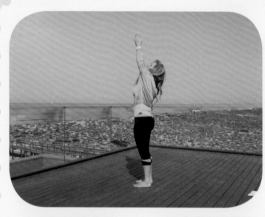

Forward Bend A
– 5 - 10 BREATHS

Hook your first two fingers around your big toes.
Keep your legs straight; if you can't straighten them, try one leg at a time. Stretch through your back and lengthen your neck.

Forward Bend B
– 5 - 10 BREATHS

Place your hands under your feet, touching your toes to the insides of your wrists.

Relax your head and breathe.

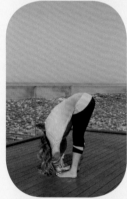
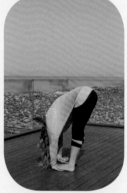

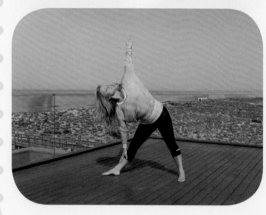

Triangle Posture – 5 - 10 BREATHS

Place your feet wide apart. Turn your right foot out and your left foot in. Stretch your arms wide and lower your right hand down towards your right ankle. Stretch your left arm up to the ceiling. Tighten your buttocks and pull up through your thighs. Look to your thumb. Repeat other side.

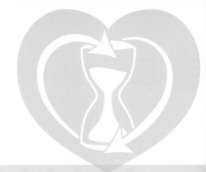

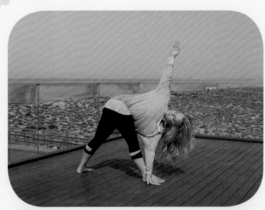

Reverse Triangle – 5 BREATHS

Start in the same position, feet wide apart. Take your right arm over to the outside of your left leg. Stretch your right arm up to the ceiling and open your chest out. Pull up through your thighs. Lift the arches of your feet. Look to your thumb. Repeat other side.

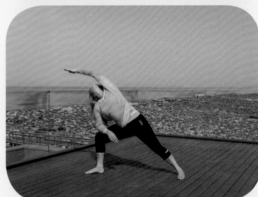

Side Flank – 5 BREATHS

Place your feet a little wider apart now. Bend your right knee and take your right elbow to your right thigh. Stretch your left arm over the side of your head, by your ear, and look to your left hand. Open chest and lift arch of left foot. Look to your thumb. Repeat other side.

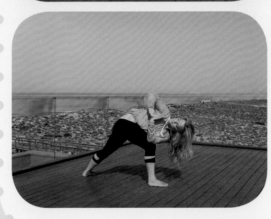

Reverse Side Flank – 5 BREATHS

Turn your right foot out and your left foot in. Take your left elbow over the outside of your right leg and place your palms together, elbows out either side. Open your chest out. Lift the arch of the left foot and pull up through that thigh. Look to the ceiling. Repeat other side.

EXERCISES
Yoga

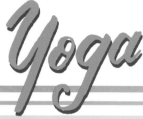

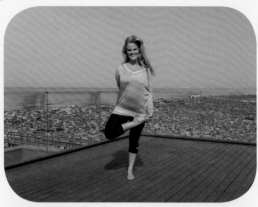

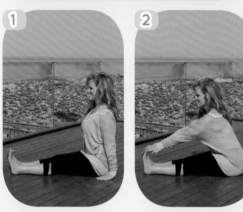

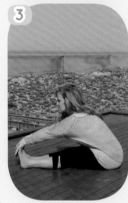

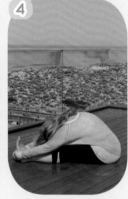

Standing Half Lotus

– 10 BREATHS

From a standing position, place your right foot on your left thigh and take your right arm behind your back, holding on to your left arm. If you can't reach your left arm, simply place your right arm behind your back. Push your right knee towards the floor. Look to the floor. Repeat other side.

Forward Bend

– 5 BREATHS EACH STEP

1 Sit with your legs straight and your feet flexed. Place your hands by your hips. Straighten through your back and pull your shoulder blades down your back. Look to your toes.

2 Hold on to your toes, pull up through your thighs, and stretch through your back. If you have to bend your knees, that's fine. Look to your toes.

3 Take your hands over the top of your feet.

4 Wrap your hands round the sides of your feet.

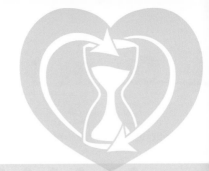

Head to Knee Forward Bend

– 5 - 10 BREATHS

Take your right foot to your left inner thigh.

Stretch your body over your thigh and reach to your left foot.

Repeat other side.

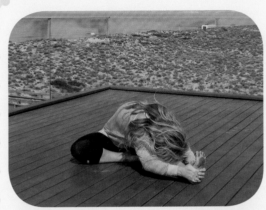

Butterfly Pose – 5 - 10 BREATHS

Sit with your feet together and your knees out to the side.

Push your knees gently in the direction of the floor.

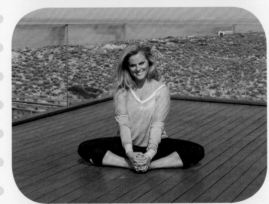

Half Lotus – 5 - 10 BREATHS

From a seated position, take your right foot to your left thigh. Flex your left foot. Hold on to your right foot with your left hand and take your right arm round behind your back; if you can, take hold of the inside of your left elbow. Look to your left foot. Repeat other side.

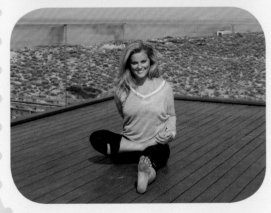

EXERCISES
Yoga

Half Lotus with Bent Knee – 5 BREATHS

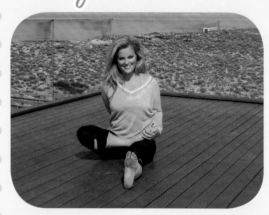

Come up from the last posture and take your left foot to your right thigh.

Repeat other side.

Back Twist – 5 - 10 BREATHS

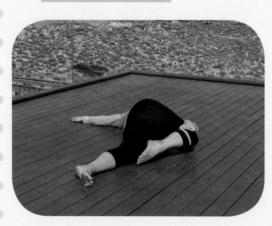

Lie on your back. Hug your right knee towards you.

Place your left hand on the outside of your right leg. Take your right arm out to the side.

Twist over so that your right knee goes to the floor and your right arm stays on the floor.

Repeat other side.

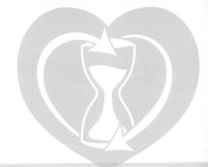

Bridge – 5 BREATHS

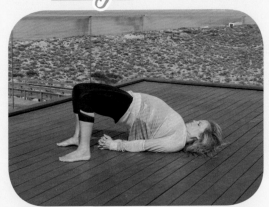

Lie on your back. Have your feet hip distance apart and raise your hips off the floor.

Squeeze your shoulder blades together and clasp your hands.

Relaxation Pose – HOLD FOR AS LONG AS YOU FEEL COMFORTABLE

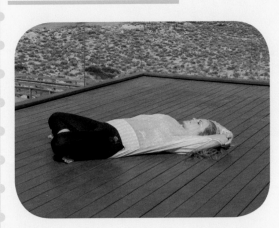

Lie on your back with your arms above your head.

Cross your legs and hold onto your elbows.

Toe Levers

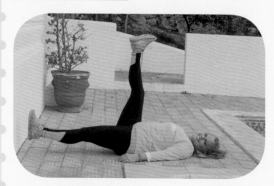

Lie on your back, raise your legs up in the air.

Lower your right leg down to the floor and then back up again, pulling your abs in. Repeat both sides.

Wall Plank

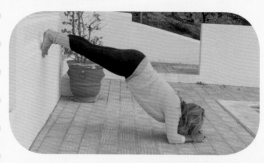

Get into plank position and then place your feet on a wall to hold your balance.

If you don't have a wall handy you can take one leg in the air and then swap over.

Remember to pull your abs in and work your core.

Oblique Wall Plank

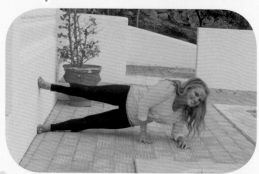

Lie on your left side and go into a side plank position.

Press your feet into the wall as you pull your abs in.

If you don't have a wall handy just raise the top leg in the air and hold. Repeat other side.

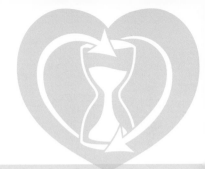

Extended Toe Levers

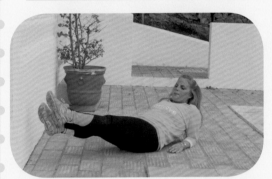

Sit down on the floor, and then rest back on your elbows, making sure your shoulders are pulled down your back.

Lower both of your legs down, breathing out as you lower, breathing in as you raise. Only go down as far as your back feels comfortable, or bend your knees if it feels like a strain on your back.

Fast Superman

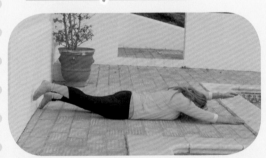

Lie on your front and raise your right arm and left leg about an inch off the floor. Look to the floor, and pull your abs in.

Now raise the left arm and right leg, lowering down the opposite. Keep repeating in a fast fashion.

Circle Abs

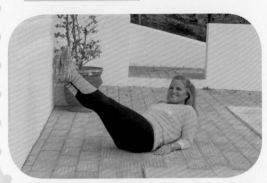

Sit down on the floor, and then rest back on your elbows, making sure your shoulders are pulled down your back. Take both legs in the air and circle your legs around, keeping your knees together.
Keep the circle small, and bend your knees if your back feels strain. Repeat other side.

	Toe Levers	Wall Plank	Oblique Wall Plank	Extended Toe Levers	Fast Superman	Circle Abs
Week 1	8	30 seconds	20 seconds, right & left	6	20	8 right, 8 left
Week 2	9	40 seconds	30 seconds, right & left	7	30	9 right, 9 left
Week 3	10	50 seconds	40 seconds, right & left	8	40	10 right, 10 left
Week 4	11	60 seconds	45 seconds, right & left	9	50	11 right, 11 left
Week 5	12	65 seconds	50 seconds, right & left	10	56	12 right, 12 left
Week 6	13	70 seconds	55 seconds, right & left	11	58	13 right, 13 left
Week 7	14	75 seconds	60 seconds, right & left	12	60	14 right, 14 left
Week 8	15	80 seconds	70 seconds, right & left	13	62	15 right, 15 left

The Body Rescue Maintenance Plan

Resistance 4

Bum-raiser — 20 RIGHT & 20 LEFT

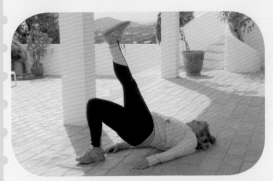

Lie on your back in bridge position. Raise your left up in the air, push through your right heel, and lift your buttocks off the floor.

Keep your left knee by the side of the right knee. Repeat, lower, and raise.

Straight Leg Bicycle — REPEAT 20 TIMES

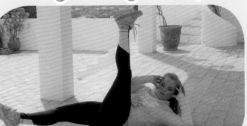

Lie on your back, take your hands to either side of your ears.

Take your left leg up in the air and take your right elbow to your left thigh, and stretch your right leg out in front of you, then change to the opposite side.

Tricep Dip Leg Raiser — REPEAT 20 RIGHT & LEFT

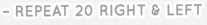

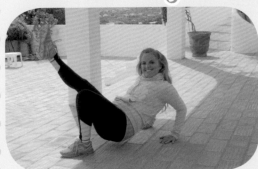

Get into a tricep dip position, lift your bottom off the floor, fingers forward, elbows back.

Raise your right leg up in the air and then bend from your elbow to lower and raise, keeping your bottom off the floor. You can also do this sitting on a chair if you wish.

Balancing Flight – HOLD FOR 1 MINUTE RIGHT, 1 MINUTE LEFT

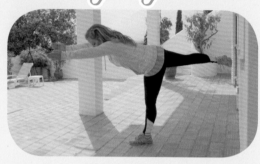

Stand with your left leg on the floor. (If you need a wall in front of you to help you with balance, or a chair, that's fine.)

Start tilting your body forward, taking your right foot off the floor. Stretch your arms out either side of you and stretch your right leg back behind you, so that your right foot is in line with your hips and shoulders, your body in one long line. Hold here, don't lock the knee, and use your core to support you, pulling your stomach in.

Isometric Extended Plank – HOLD FOR 1 MINUTE

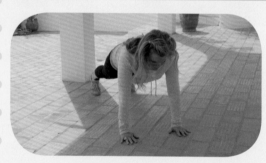

Place your hands on the floor in an extended plank position, with your legs straight, knees off the floor.

Push through your heels and have your shoulder blades down your back. Pull your stomach in. Hold this position, working the core, pulling the abs in.

Side Lunge into Lateral Raise – 20 RIGHT & 20 LEFT

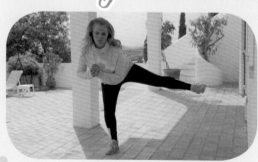

Go into a side lunge position, left leg extended to the side, right knee bent into a squat.

Now raise up from the squat and raise your left leg into the air, and then repeat.

Interval 4

DO EACH EXERCISE FOR 20 SECONDS, THEN HAVE A 10 SECOND REST.
ALL 8 EXERCISES EQUAL 1 ROUND; DO 4 ROUNDS.

Lunge Box

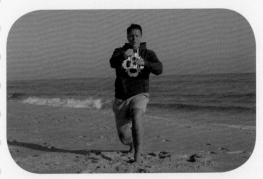

Step forward into a lunge position with your left leg; take your right leg behind you and lunge down. Take your hands to your chest and punch left and right as if you are hitting pads in front of you. As you do this, pull in from your core. Repeat on the other side in the next round.

Extended Plank Arm Pull

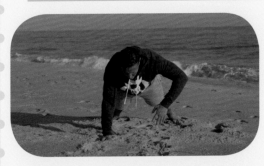

Go into an extended plank position, the wider your legs are the easier it is, choose a position to suit you.

Pull your abs in, breathe out and raise your right hand to your right armpit, and then lower again. Repeat this side. Begin the other side on the next round.

Squat Punch

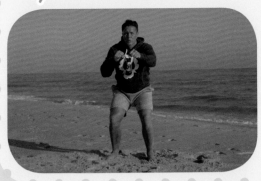

Go into a squat position, bending your knees and sticking your bottom out, like you are about to sit down. Feet are forward-facing and hip distance apart.

Stay in a squat and punch upwards towards the ceiling, no higher than your chin; pull in from the abs, and push down through your heels.

Squat & Twist

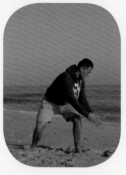 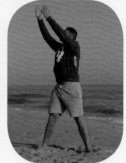

Squat down and twist towards your left foot, reaching your arms down to the floor.

Now stand up and rise up as if you are holding a ball, taking your arms up above your right shoulder, and twisting the other way. Repeat. Do the other side the next round.

Tuck Jumps

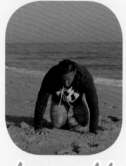 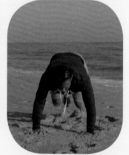

Go into an extended plank position, and jump both feet towards your chest and then back again.

If the jumping is too difficult for you then step alternate legs in, keep your bottom low.

Lunge Hops

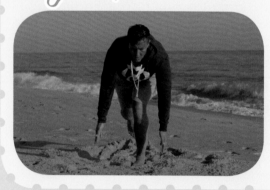

Go into a lunge position with your right leg forwards, and then raise your left leg off the floor, and lean forwards with your arms in a skater position.

Leap up in the air and land with your left leg on the floor and your right leg behind you, Keep repeating.

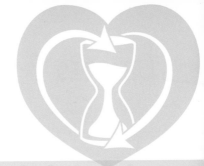

Wide Angle Squat Jump

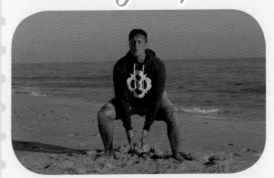

Bend your knees in a squat, with your feet turned outwards and your legs wider than your hips.

Jump up in the air and land again, bending down. Keep your back up tall, and look forwards, not down.

Extended Plank, Elbow to Knee

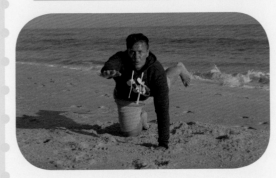

Go into the extended plank position and extend your right arm and left leg straight out, then take your right elbow to your left knee.

Keep repeating this side and then do the other side on the next round. Keep your hips as low as possible. Pull your abs in.

Yoga

CONTINUE THE SAME AS BE-

EXERCISES
Abs 5

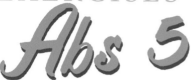

DO EVERYDAY

Lever Cycles

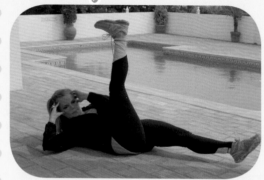

Lie on your back. Lift your head and shoulders and raise your feet off the floor a few inches. If this feels like too much pressure on your back, bend your knees a little or raise your legs higher towards you.

Now raise your back off the floor, sitting up and at the same time bend your right knee towards you, taking your left elbow towards your right knee, and your right elbow to your right waist. Lower back down carefully, breathing out, and then repeat the other side.

Plank Elbow to Knee

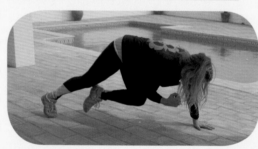

Go into the extended plank position and extend your right arm and left leg straight out, then take your right elbow to your left knee.

Keep repeating this side and then do the other side on the next round. Keep your hips as low as possible. Pull your abs in.

Oblique Swings

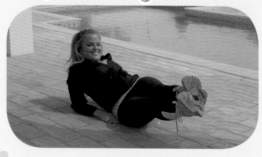

Sit on the floor. Rest your forearms on the floor, with your fingers pointing forward.

Bend your knees and then roll onto your right hip, extending your legs. Bend your knees in again and then repeat to the other side.

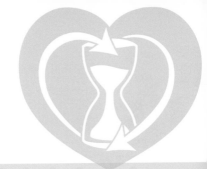

Toe Touches

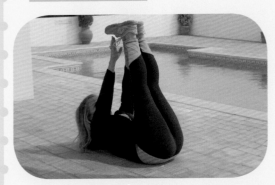

Lie on your back with your legs extended to the ceiling. Raise your head and shoulders off the floor, reaching your arms to your feet.

Keep your middle back as high up as possible, and touch your fingers to your toes, tapping. Move 1 inch forwards and back.

Frontal Levers

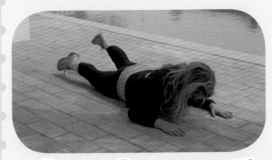

Lie on your front.

Lift your chest and head off the floor, keeping your forearms on the floor.

Raise alternate legs.

Seated Balancing Twists

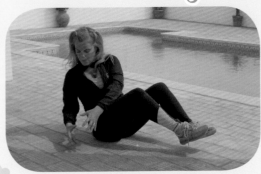

From a seated position, lift your feet off the floor, knees bent.

Either hold a ball or place your hands in that position, and twist from your torso so the ball is over the right hip, with your body in alignment, then twist to the other side, balancing with your feet off the floor.

	Lever Cycles	Plank Elbow to Knee	Oblique Swings	Toe Touches	Frontal Levers	Seated Balancing Twists
Week 1	2 sets of 6	16 right & left	6	50	20	20
Week 2	2 sets of 8	18 right & left	8	60	22	22
Week 3	2 sets of 10	20 right & left	10	70	24	24
Week 4	2 sets of 12	22 right & left	12	80	26	26
Week 5	2 sets of 14	24 right & left	14	80	28	28
Week 6	2 sets of 16	26 right & left	18	90	30	30
Week 7	2 sets of 18	28 right & left	20	100	32	32
Week 8	2 sets of 20	30 right & left	22	110	34	34

The Body Rescue Maintenance Plan

Resistance 5

One-legged Bum Raise – 20 RIGHT & 20 LEFT

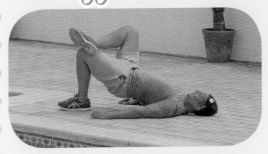

Lie in a bridge position, take your arms out straight, shoulders down the back.

Take your right foot over your left thigh. Push through your left heel and raise and lower the hips.

Waist Slimmers – 2 SETS OF 16

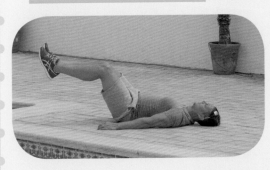

Lie on your back with your legs in the air and your arms out to the sides.

Lower your legs to the left, pulling in through the core. Raise up again, to the ceiling, then lower to the right. Try not to push in through your arms too much. If it's too difficult you can bend your knees a little.

Ballet Shoot – HOLD FOR 30 SECONDS RIGHT & LEFT

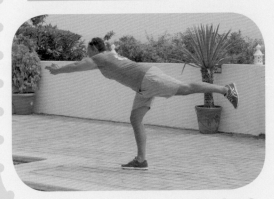

From a standing position, take your right leg off the floor and stretch it back behind you. At the same time, stretch both your arms together in front of you, holding your hands in the shoot position.

If you are finding it hard to balance, use a wall in front of you to hold yourself initially. Do not lock your standing leg.

EXERCISES
Resistance 5

One-legged Bridge — 20 RIGHT & 20 LEFT

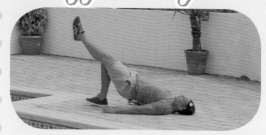

Lie in a bridge position and raise your left leg in the air, with your arms straight by your sides.

Keep your leg extended to the ceiling and lower and raise the hips.

Narrow & Wide Press-ups — 2 SETS OF 12

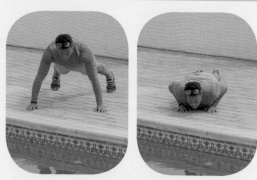

In an extended plank position, have your hands and feet narrow, shoulder width apart. Now bend at the elbows, keeping your elbows to your waist. If this is too hard, take your knees on the floor and try from a half press-up position.

Push back up again and this time take your arms and legs wide and press down again. Repeat.

Open Side Plank — 20 RIGHT & 20 LEFT

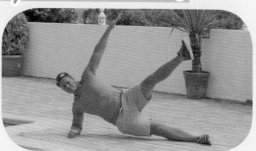

Start in a side plank position on your right arm, with your left hand to your hip. Now raise your left arm and left leg in the air and then bring them back down again.

If this is too difficult, put your left hand on the floor supporting you and just try raising the leg initially. For an advanced move, do it continually.
To make it easier, lower the hip down and then raise up again between each rep.

Interval 5

DO EACH EXERCISE FOR 20 SECONDS, THEN HAVE A 10 SECOND REST. ALL 8 EXERCISES EQUAL 1 ROUND; DO 4 ROUNDS.

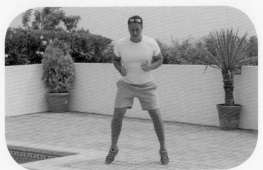

Inner & Outer Drills

Run on the spot at a fast pace for 10, then open your legs wide and run fast for 10.

If your body does not like running, then walk fast instead.

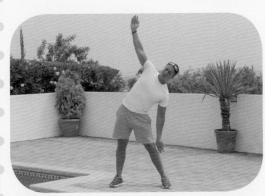

Triangle Waist Levers

Stand with your feet over hip distance apart, toes pointing forward. Raise your left arm up to the ceiling and lower your right hand down to the right ankle.

Keeping your arms apart, lift up to a standing position again and then lower down again. Repeat on the right then change to the other side on the next round.

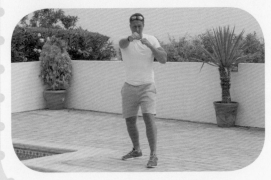

Boxing

From a standing position box as fast as you can, punching the air in front of your chest, whilst clenching your fists.

EXERCISES
Interval 5

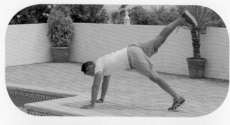

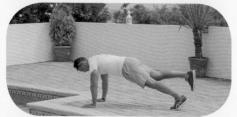

Dolphin Dive

From an extended plank position, raise your right leg up in the air behind you, stretching it back as far as you can.

Then lower your hips down towards the floor, not letting your back arch, and not touching the floor, then lift back up again.

Do the right leg this round and change sides the next.

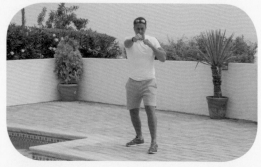

Slow Boxing

This time punch slowly, breathing out sharply as you punch, and pulling your whole core area in; keep your legs bent at the knee.

Butt Squeeze

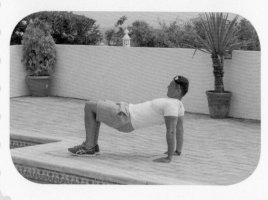

Sit on the floor and place your hands on the floor, fingers forward.

Raise your hips off the floor, to shoulder height, then lower back down again. Squeeze your buttocks as you do this.

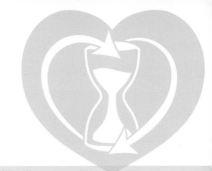

Side Lunge to Squat

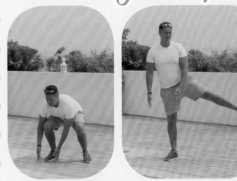

From a standing position, step your left leg out to the left side and squat right down, keeping your head up and stretching your right left out to the side, your arms either side of your left foot.

If you can, reach to the floor. Repeat other side, push through the heel of the leg that is squatting.

Lower Leg Side Plank

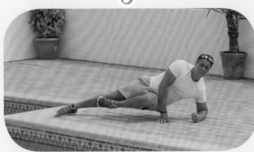

Lie on your left side in a side plank, with your left forearm on the floor. Take your right hand to your right hip and hold it there.

Bring your left knee up towards your chest, keeping your body long and repeat. Do the right side the next round.

Yoga

CONTINUE THE SAME AS BE-

Memberships

Why not choose one of our award-winning membership plans to help you on your weight loss journey? Go to:

WWW.THEBODYRESCUEPLAN.COM

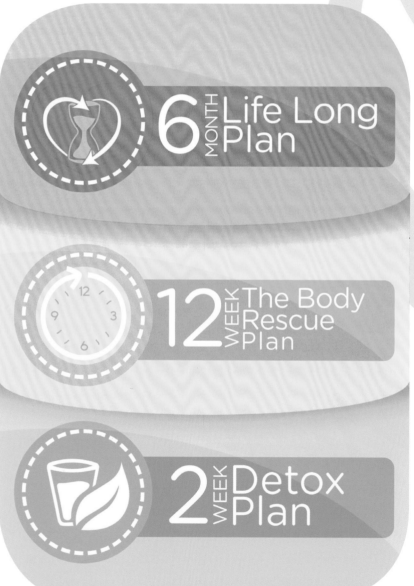

6 MONTH Life Long Plan

12 WEEK The Body Rescue Plan

2 WEEK Detox Plan

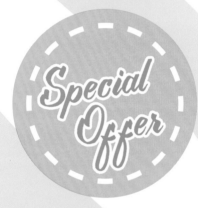

Special Offer

Use this discount code for **50% off** the first month of the Maintenance membership, simply add the coupon code:

Maintainyourlife

at the checkout!

Download Your Free Meditation CD Now!

To download your **FREE meditation CD** please go to the following page:
WWW.THEBODYRESCUEPLAN.COM/MEDITATION-AUDIO-REQUEST/
and enter the code:

TBRP1

or for your gratitude meditations enter the code:

TBRMP1

Please note you cannot download directly onto a phone or iPad. To get the meditations onto your phone or iPad you can download to iTunes using your computer and then they can be uploaded from there to your phone or iPad.

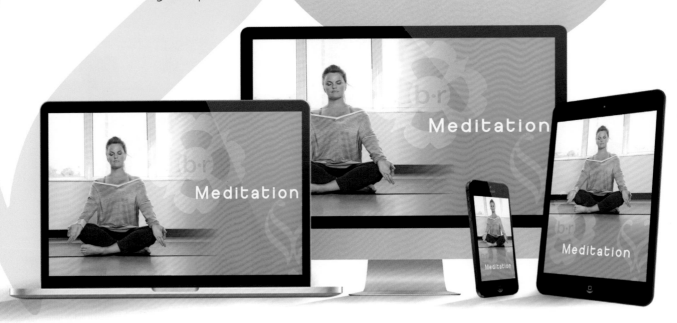

bodyrescue
SLIMMING CLUBS UK

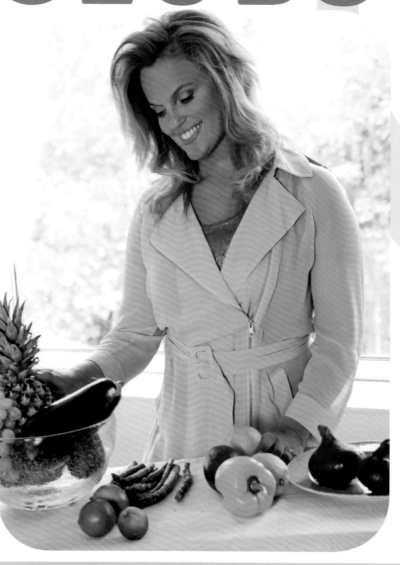
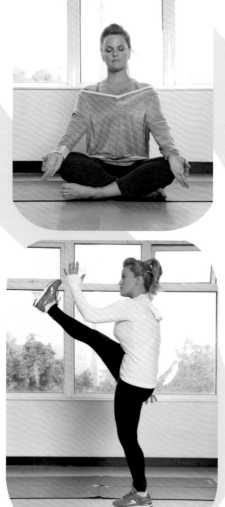

The Body Rescue Maintenance Plan

Coming Soon!

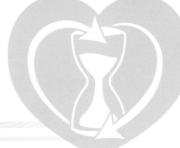

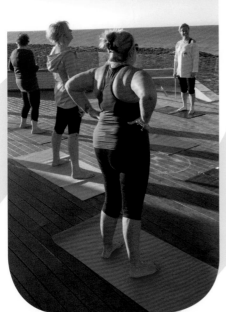

The Body Rescue Slimming Clubs will be starting around the UK from January 2017. If you would like support from your local Body Rescue coach, and to be part of these award-winning classes then go to www.thebodyrescueplan.com to find out more.

If you are interested in becoming a franchisee and owning your own Body Rescue Slimming Club, then contact our team on info@ bodyrescue.net for more details or go to www.thebodyrescueplan.com

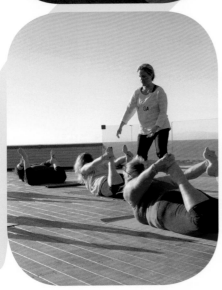

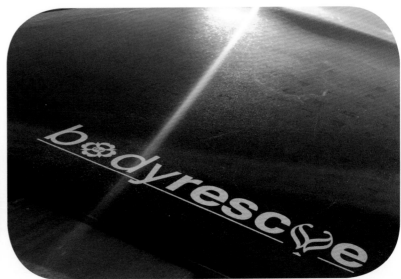

Good luck with your journey and keep in touch on my social media sites!

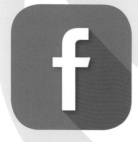
The Body Rescue Plan

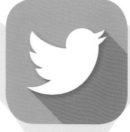
Christianne_w

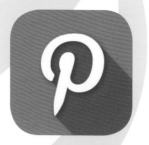
Christianne Wolff

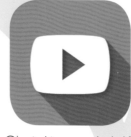
Christianne Wolff

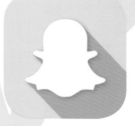
Christianne_w

Or why not check out our amazing fitness retreats around the world:

WWW.THEBODYRESCUEPLAN/FITNESS-RETREATS/

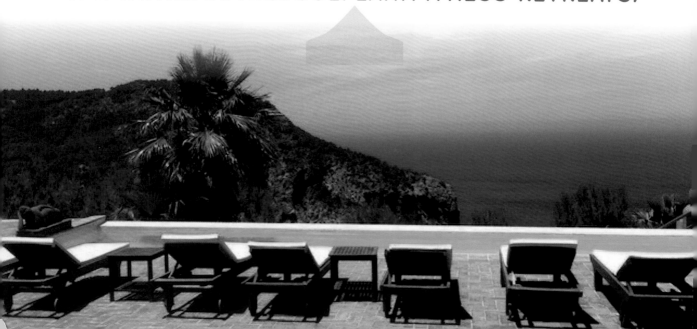